Why Women Need Fat

Why Women Need Fat

How "Healthy" Food Makes Us Gain
Excess Weight and the Surprising
Solution to Losing It Forever

**William D. Lassek, M.D.
and Steven J. C. Gaulin, Ph.D.**

HUDSON
STREET
PRESS

HUDSON STREET PRESS
Published by Penguin Group
Penguin Group (USA) Inc., 375 Hudson Street, New York, New York 10014, U.S.A. • Penguin Group (Canada), 90 Eglinton Avenue East, Suite 700, Toronto, Ontario, Canada M4P 2Y3 (a division of Pearson Penguin Canada Inc.) • Penguin Books Ltd., 80 Strand, London WC2R 0RL, England • Penguin Ireland, 25 St. Stephen's Green, Dublin 2, Ireland (a division of Penguin Books Ltd.) • Penguin Group (Australia), 250 Camberwell Road, Camberwell, Victoria 3124, Australia (a division of Pearson Australia Group Pty. Ltd.) • Penguin Books India Pvt. Ltd., 11 Community Centre, Panchsheel Park, New Delhi – 110 017, India • Penguin Books (NZ), 67 Apollo Drive, Rosedale, Auckland 0632, New Zealand (a division of Pearson New Zealand Ltd.) • Penguin Books (South Africa) (Pty.) Ltd., 24 Sturdee Avenue, Rosebank, Johannesburg 2196, South Africa

Penguin Books Ltd., Registered Offices: 80 Strand, London WC2R 0RL, England

First published by Hudson Street Press, a member of Penguin Group (USA) Inc.

First Printing, January 2012
10 9 8 7 6 5 4 3 2 1

REGISTERED TRADEMARK—MARCA REGISTRADA
HUDSON
STREET
PRESS

LIBRARY OF CONGRESS CATALOGING-IN-PUBLICATION DATA

Lassek, William D.
  Why women need fat : how "healthy" food makes us gain excess weight and the surprising solution to losing it forever / William D. Lassek and Steven J. C. Gaulin.
     p. cm.
  Includes bibliographical references and index.
  ISBN 978-1-59463-085-9 (hardback)
  1. Women—Nutrition.   2. Women—Health and hygiene.   3. Lipids in human nutrition.
4. Weight loss.   I. Gaulin, Steven J. C.   II. Title.
  RA778.L354 2011
  613'.04244—dc23
                                                                                            2011029757

Printed in the United States of America
Set in Bembo Std

PUBLISHER'S NOTE
Every effort has been made to ensure that the information contained in this book is complete and accurate. However, neither the publisher nor the authors are engaged in rendering professional advice or services to the individual reader. The ideas, procedures, and suggestions contained in this book are not intended as a substitute for consulting with your physician. All matters regarding your health require medical supervision. Neither the authors nor the publisher shall be liable or responsible for any loss or damage allegedly arising from any information or suggestion in this book.

While the authors have made every effort to provide accurate telephone numbers and Internet addresses at the time of publication, neither the publisher nor the authors assume any responsibility for errors, or for changes that occur after publication. Further, the publisher does not have any control over and does not assume any responsibility for author or third-party Web sites or their content.

ALWAYS LEARNING   PEARSON

This book is dedicated to the many wonderful women in our lives—mothers, partners, sisters, daughters, and granddaughters—and to all American women in their ongoing quest for better lives for themselves and their loved ones.

ACKNOWLEDGMENTS

Many people have helped inspire and shape this book. Many of the ideas in it are new, and our mentors, colleagues, and students have all asked the right questions at key junctures. But still, a smaller number of people made such clear and identifiable contributions that we must mention them by name.

As some of the ideas in this book were coalescing, we benefited greatly from thoughtful questioning by the faculty and doctoral students of the Center for Evolutionary Psychology and the Integrative Anthropological Sciences Program at the University of California, Santa Barbara. There, Melanie Martin, Mike Gurven, John Tooby, Leda Cosmides, Jim Roney, Daniel Sznycer, Carolyn Hodges, Kate Hanson, Max Krasnow, Andy Delton, Tess Robertson, and Danielle Truxaw were especially helpful.

It was Melanie who carefully collected breast milk among the Tsimane people of Amazonian Bolivia, guarded it within liquid nitrogen, and navigated it through customs. We thank those Tsimane mothers for their contributions, and Rhob Evans at the University of Pittsburgh's Graduate School of Public Health for his time and expertise in analyzing the fatty acids in their milk and the comparison sample from

American mothers provided by Ardith Morrow, Jessica Woo, Barbara S. Davidson, and Sheela R. Geraghty.

Colleagues elsewhere—in particular, Dan Fessler, Martie Haselton, Caleb Finch, Roberta Ness, and Joseph Hibbeln—brought their own special expertise to bear in helping us refine our thinking. A lineage of astute research assistants, including Natalie Brechtel, Aimée K. Andrews, Liana Hone, and Aymee Fenwick, measured, weighed, and pinched many an obliging young woman or helped scour federal government databases. We also wish to thank Donna Bushey and Joanna Saykiewicz for their valuable help. Will especially thanks his best friend and companion of many years, Mary Carrasco, for her support and uniformly good advice.

Norm Lee and the family of our late colleague Professor Devendra Singh—especially his daughter Dorian Singh—generously shared their recollections of Dev and how he came to launch an area of research that now spans the biological and social sciences. Likewise, we are grateful to Dr. Ulf Högberg for the story of why he undertook research on deaths from childbirth in nineteenth-century Sweden.

Kate Lee, our agent at ICM, saw what this project could be perhaps more fully than we did; and our editors at the Penguin Group—Caroline Sutton and Meghan Stevenson—did much to help the vision become a reality. This book would not exist without the energies and insights of these three dynamic women. We would also like to thank copy editor Sheila Moody and managing editor Norina Frabotta.

None of these generous people are to blame for any errors we have made or wrong turnings we may have taken.

Finally, we are grateful to the thousands of women and their daughters (as well as the men and boys) who have willingly participated in the National Health and Nutrition Examination Surveys conducted by the U.S. Public Health Service over the past fifty years. They have generously shared their exhaustive histories, measurements, habits, bodily fluids, X-rays, and dietary choices with medical researchers. Without their unsung sacrifices, so important to this book, the health of Americans would be much less well understood and our efforts to improve it much diminished.

CONTENTS

INTRODUCTION

S usan is a pretty typical American woman. She's a forty-five-year-old divorcée, has a daughter and a son, works as the manager of a church-based nursery school, and would very much like to lose weight. Her height (five feet, four inches) and weight (166 pounds) are close to the average for American women her age. Her body mass index (BMI) is 28, near the upper end of the "overweight" range. Even though Susan is currently in good health, her doctor has told her that she is substantially overweight and should really try to lose at least ten pounds, pointing out that being overweight can increase fat and sugar in her blood, make her white blood cells more active, and raise her blood pressure.

Unfortunately, being told she should lose weight isn't doing Susan any good. She has been trying to lose weight for most of the past twenty years and has tried just about every kind of diet plan or program imaginable. With each one, she usually has some initial success and once even lost twenty-five pounds. But typically, after she loses ten or fifteen pounds, her weight loss stops. Even worse, although she usually tries to maintain her diet, she not only regains the lost weight but ends up gaining more. The net result is that, despite all of her efforts to lose weight, she has gained seventeen pounds in the last ten years.

What makes this all the more painful for Susan is that in her late teens and early twenties, she was not only thin but it was easy for her to stay that way. On the day she graduated from high school, she weighed 118 pounds, and until she became pregnant with her daughter Jessica when she was twenty-three, she stayed close to 120 pounds without any effort and without dieting, special exercise, or feeling hungry. Back then she had an hourglass figure with a narrow waist and rounded hips and thighs. Based on her height and weight at that time, she would have had about thirty-five pounds of fat—about half of what she has now.

But after her daughter was born, Susan never got back to her old weight, and her weight crept up even more after she had her son David. Despite her frequent dieting, every year she gained one or two pounds, until one day she realized that she had gained almost fifty pounds since her high school graduation day. As her mother likes to remind her, she now weighs twenty pounds more than her mother did at the same age. Susan often wonders how that slender nineteen-year-old became a forty-five-year-old woman who is twenty-one pounds overweight with nearly seventy pounds of body fat. It's a common question among American women and it's what we are going to try to answer in this book.

Susan's Story Is the Story of Most Women

Not all women gain as much as Susan has and, certainly, some gain more. But Susan's experience of starting out thin and then steadily gaining weight after having children is the story of most women around the world. As was true for Susan before she became a mom, most young women who have not been pregnant tend to be thin, typically weighing around 120 pounds if they have an average height of five feet, four inches. (For taller or shorter women, each inch in height adds or subtracts about five pounds.) These low weights have been typical for women in their late teens in countries all around the world and, until the 1970s, were true of most young American women as well.

After starting out thin, as Susan did, most women (who live where there is enough to eat) tend to gain weight in their childbearing years, adding about a pound a year as they raise their families. Susan's mom went through this, gaining twenty-five pounds and weighing 146 by her late forties. From the time when average weights began to be tabulated, in the 1890s, until the 1970s, American women showed this same pattern of moderate weight gain. (Men do not gain in this way; they typically add less weight from their twenties to their forties.)

We can also see that same pattern in women gaining weight if we look further back in time: In paintings from past centuries, maidens are usually slim, while mothers with children are heavier. So, everywhere there is enough food—including the United States up until the 1970s—women typically start out at around 120 pounds in their late teens, gain about one pound a year, and weigh around 145 pounds by their mid-forties. Even though American women now weigh more than they used to, almost two-thirds of their weight gain is typical of women in the past and is still normal for women in European countries. So part of the answer to Susan's question lies in understanding why women normally gain weight; explaining this will be our focus in part 2.

However, something has definitely changed for American women in the past forty years. They have been gaining more weight than they did in the past, and many have become unhappy participants in our "obesity epidemic." Just as Susan weighs more than her mother did at her age, the average American woman today weighs twenty pounds more than her counterpart did forty years ago or than the average woman in Europe does today. Back in the early 1970s, only one American woman in seven was considered "obese" (with a BMI of 30 or more); now twice as many (more than one in three) fall into this group.

Because many women weigh more now, it's not surprising that, like Susan, so many are trying to lose weight. Three out of four American women would like to weigh less than they do; and most of them have tried to lose weight during the past year, spending more than *$40 billion* on diet books, special foods, and weight-loss programs. However, despite their determined efforts and painful sacrifices, half of those trying to lose ended up gaining weight by the end of the year, with a third of those who tried to lose gaining more than five pounds. In chapter 7 we will explain why dieting is a leading cause of weight *gain*.

While young American women in the past and young women in other countries today have usually been thin before having children, as Susan was in her early twenties, that, too, has been changing. Susan's twenty-two-year-old daughter Jessica already weighs 145 pounds, typical of American women her age today who have not had children and twenty pounds heavier than her mom or grandmother at the same age. The number of *young* women above "normal" weight has almost tripled since 1970 to one in two, and the rate of "obesity" in this age group has increased fourfold, to one in four.

Children—both girls and boys—also seem to be gaining weight at an alarming pace. The proportion considered overweight has more than doubled to one in three and the number who are obese has increased almost fourfold to one in five. We don't know for certain what will happen to these heavier young women and girls as they get older, but if they experience the same weight gain as their mothers, *two-thirds* of today's young American women will become obese as they age. We will be focusing on the reasons for these alarming increases in weight in part 1 and the remedies in part 3.

Susan and Jessica are typical examples of what is happening to many American women, raising two puzzling questions. Why do women normally start out thin and gain weight as they age? And, critically, why are American women gaining much more weight than their counterparts around the world? The answers to these questions not only help make sense of women's unique biology, but also point to how sensible diet and lifestyle choices can lead to more natural, healthy weights for women and their children.

How We Came to Write This Book

It would be nice to say that we started out with a set of straightforward and logically connected questions about women's weights and then set out to answer them in a systematic and orderly fashion, but that's not what happened. When we started working together, we were not thinking at all about why women gain weight or why American women have recently been gaining more. Instead, we were trying to answer an entirely different question: why men find women's hourglass figures attractive. This question had already been puzzling a lot of folks in academia. So in 2003, we decided to join our different skills together to study it.

Steve is a professor of anthropology at the University of California, Santa Barbara. He trained in both anthropology and psychology and for the past ten years he has been co–editor in chief of *Evolution and Human Behavior*, the leading scientific journal looking at the connections between evolution, anthropology, and psychology.

He has devoted his career to helping to pioneer a new field called *evolutionary psychology*, a discipline aimed at discovering the ancient roots of some of our distinctively human patterns of thinking and behaving. This field is based on the simple idea that whatever qualities helped people to have more and healthier children in the past would have been passed down to the present in our genes. From this perspective, the question is always *why* we are the way we are and how it helped our ancestors to survive and reproduce.

Steve's main research focus has been on why male and female animals—and, more interestingly, men and women—differ. For example, he and his colleagues found that women do better than men at remembering the location of cards in a memory game. But why would this be useful? In groups who still live as our hunter-gatherer ancestors did during the Stone Age, women are responsible for gathering plant foods; so remembering where they are is essential for them. Since men hunt animals that roam around, remembering particular locations isn't so useful for them. This suggests that women should be especially good at remembering where they have seen edible plants; sure enough, women are better than men at remembering where fruits and vegetables are in a farmers' market, especially those with the most calories. Steve's approach, which looks at the ancient roots of our biology and behavior, will help us uncover the underlying reasons women need fat and why we're getting fatter.

Will's path was quite different. He began his career working as a U.S. Public Health Service physician in a remote Eskimo village in northwestern Alaska, followed by work in obstetrics and at a women's health clinic in New York City. He became increasingly interested in trying to understand the cause of differences in health between various groups of people, and he eventually became an assistant surgeon general. He is currently an assistant professor of epidemiology at the University of Pittsburgh's Graduate School of Public Health and a research associate in the Department of Anthropology at the University of California, Santa Barbara.

Medicine has a set of questions very different from anthropology's; physicians don't usually ask *why* we are the way we are, as anthropologists do. In medical practice, we begin with a patient who has particular symptoms, like the sudden severe pain in the chest and left arm that often signals a heart attack. We then try to understand why our patient has those symptoms so that we can do something to help. In this case, we usually find that people have this kind of chest pain when one of the coronary arteries that supplies blood to the heart is blocked by a blood clot, and we can treat this blockage with drugs that dissolve the clot or with surgery.

In public health, on the other hand, we step back to look at groups of patients, such as the group who have had heart attacks. When we ask how they differ from others, we find that heart attack victims are more likely to have certain "risk factors" like elevated blood pressure or cholesterol in the blood, or smoking. We can also use this same public health approach to look at groups of people who may be at greater risk for health problems, such as those with a BMI over 30 (designated as "obese") who may be more likely to have heart attacks or strokes than those who are less heavy.

When we look further, we find that heavier people tend to have higher levels of blood pressure, fat and sugar in the blood, and white blood cell activity—just as Susan's doctor has told her—and these factors may increase their chances of developing blood vessel disease. But this is usually where we stop in medicine and public health. We don't go one step further and ask *why* women with a higher weight have more of these factors, *why* the two are linked. But the answer to the question why turns out to be a very fruitful question for a partnership between a physician and an anthropologist.

We first met when Will sat in on a course Steve was teaching, called "Sex and Evolution," and made a nuisance of himself by asking lots of complicated questions that confused Steve's students. But when Steve learned about Will's background in medicine and public health, he asked Will to work with him on the question of why men find the smaller waists and larger hips typical of young women attractive. This was a question that had attracted the attention of many anthropologists and psychologists, especially those interested in how evolution might have shaped our minds. The basic idea is that men should prefer mates who will help them have more and healthier children. So how does attractiveness—specifically, a woman's body shape—predict her future success as a mother? And if it doesn't, why should men care?

The prevailing view was that women who have smaller waists in relation to their hips—a smaller "waist-hip ratio"—have better health and higher fertility. Many medical studies have looked at how this ratio relates to health. By putting our two different viewpoints together, we wanted to go deeper. We wondered just *why* having a smaller waist and larger hips might help a woman to have more and healthier children. What could be the physical connection between a woman's body shape and her success as a mother? Our attempts to solve this mystery, related in part 2, eventually led us, through many twists and turns, to Susan's question.

Three Puzzles

We tackle three puzzling questions in this book: why typical young women start out with the low weights and low waist-hip ratios that men admire; why these same women add fat as they get older; and why American women like Susan and Jessica are heavier now than they were forty years ago.

Each of these questions reflects a part of Susan's experience. Like most young women, she started out relatively slender. Her current weight is the result of both the normal gain all mothers experience and the upward climb of American women's weights that began about forty years ago. So, to fully answer Susan's question about her weight, we need to solve all of these puzzles.

In part 1 we look at how changes in the American diet intended to make us healthier have led women to gain much more weight than they did in the past; in part 2 we focus on why women's figures change as they grow older and have children.

In part 3 we look at how women can use our results to find their natural healthy weight and body type. Although American women are heavier today than they used to be, they don't have to be. From why dieting doesn't work to specific suggestions about which foods and beverages are best, we will give advice on how a woman like Susan or Jessica can recover her lower natural weight.

Our Goals

If women can understand the reasons why their bodies need to gain weight after a first child and why this is beneficial, it may be easier to accept that keeping the slender figure of their youth may not be possible or even desirable. We believe that knowledge and understanding are always empowering, especially when some of the lessons contradict long-held ideals.

Understanding why they need fat can also help women to take steps to have the right amount and the right kind. The reasons women are heavier than they used to be are strongly connected to why women have extra fat in the first place and to why this fat changes when they have children. As we uncover these relationships, we can identify a pattern of dietary and lifestyle choices that can help counter the excessive weight gains that have become common for many in the last few decades.

How This Book Is Organized

There are three components to this book that readers may find helpful: chapters, notes, and appendix. The notes section is keyed to the page numbers in the chapters. To find out more about something you read on a page in a chapter, you can look for that page number in the notes. Many of the ideas in this book are new and unfamiliar and are based on our own research, and we provide the sources we used for our original research in an authors' note preceding the notes section. The authors' note also has our analysis of new fatty acid data for American women, which became available too late to include in the chapters but which strongly supports many of the key ideas in this book. The notes section also includes many references from the scientific literature that supports our ideas. The appendix has more detailed information in the form of tables and may be of interest to a reader who would like more specifics. It includes information on the fats that are an important part of our story and specific foods that influence weight gain. We will now start our journey with the strange story of how changes in the American diet intended to make us healthy made us fat instead.

Part One

Why and How We Got Fatter

CHAPTER 1

Why Our Diet Changed

L ike most American women, Susan is the one in her family who usually shops for food, plans the meals, and prepares them. Because she is largely responsible for deciding on the foods that she and her family will eat and she wants everyone to be healthy, she tries to choose foods that she believes will foster good health. To help her do this, she reads the nutrition information and ingredient lists on the labels of processed or packaged foods. She pays particular attention to the amount of total and saturated fat and the number of calories per serving. And she's also familiar with the national *Dietary Guidelines* and its "food pyramid," which proclaims that fat—especially saturated fat—is supposed to be bad for us, while polyunsaturated fat is thought to be better.

Since every processed or packaged food that we buy has a label detailing its fat content, you would think that there must be no doubt that these fats have a strong impact on our health. Surely there must be strong scientific evidence that following these dietary recommendations will improve our health. We know, for example, that if you have high blood pressure, taking medication to lower it can help you live longer. We know this because medical studies have shown it to be true. We also know that having mammograms can reduce deaths from breast cancer in women over fifty because studies have shown that they do. If women didn't believe that there was good evidence that it was beneficial, they certainly wouldn't do it. So surely there must be many medical studies showing that following recommendations to change the fats in your diet will make you healthier.

But surprisingly, astoundingly, there aren't. There are *no* credible studies that show that following the recommendations to reduce total and saturated fat while increasing polyunsaturated fat will make you healthier. In 1993, physicians began enrolling more than forty-eight thousand middle-aged American women in the most recent of many studies investigating the health benefits of changing fat in the diet in accordance with the goals long enshrined in our *Dietary Guidelines.* Half of the women were given intensive training and assistance to help them to decrease the total fat and saturated fat in their diets to levels even lower than those in our national goals. The other half were left alone to eat whatever they wanted.

The women with the intensive diet advice did remarkably well in changing their diets. They decreased the total fat, saturated fat, and cholesterol in their diets by a *third* while increasing the proportion of polyunsaturated fat. Their total fat and saturated fat intakes were well below the levels that the national goals and food labels aim for, just as the researchers had hoped they would be. They did even better than what the guidelines ask us to do. And the cholesterol in their blood did decrease by a small amount. Meanwhile, the women in the comparison group did not change their diets, and their cholesterol stayed the same.

After eight years had passed, the researchers looked at how many women in the two groups had suffered heart attacks or strokes or had died from either cause. They had expected that women who had changed their diets so dramatically would do much better than those who had not. But there was *no difference* in the number of heart attacks, strokes, or deaths between the women who had changed their diets and the women who had not changed. Changing dietary fat even more than our national goals call for made absolutely no difference to whether they had a heart attack or stroke or died from one.

But this is only one of many studies with the same negative results.

In the famous Framingham Heart Study, for example, which followed more than five thousand residents of a Massachusetts town for thirty years, there was *no relationship* between what people ate and whether they developed heart disease or died prematurely, and many other studies have also found no effect. One recent review analyzed twenty-one different studies and concluded that there was *no evidence* that saturated fat in the diet increases the risk of heart attacks or strokes. Another review found an astonishing lack of scientific evidence supporting any of the current recommendations in the *Dietary Guidelines.*

So how did we come to have dietary guidelines, national goals, food pyramids, and food labels telling us to change our diets and eat less of some fats and more of others if there were no studies showing that making these changes would make us healthier? It turns out that two men were largely responsible for bringing about the remarkable changes in the American diet: one who could not have been more eager to lead the charge, and one who would much rather not have been involved at all.

Ike's Multibillion-Dollar Heart Attack

On a pleasant fall afternoon in September 1955, the thirty-fourth president of the United States, Dwight Eisenhower, then sixty-four, was playing a lackluster round of golf. His stomach was bothering him; could it have been that onion-laden hamburger he'd eaten for lunch? He tried to ignore his discomfort and kept playing. But a few hours after going to bed that evening, he awakened with a severe pain in his chest and asked his wife, Mamie, to bring him some milk of magnesia. After one look at him, Mamie insisted that they call his doctor, and tests soon showed that he had suffered a major heart attack caused by a clot blocking one of the coronary arteries that supplied blood to his heart.

Ike then made a fateful and courageous decision. Though he would be running for reelection the following year and his opponents were sure to make his health an issue, he decided to tell the American public exactly what had happened. The news that the country's beloved president, the hero who had won the war against the Nazis, had suffered a serious heart attack sent a shock wave through the country. The stock market suffered its largest loss to date—shedding $14 billion in a single day—and the American public instantly developed a voracious appetite for information about coronary arteries, atherosclerosis, and cholesterol.

Fortunately, the famous Boston heart specialist brought in to take charge of the president's case, Dr. Paul Dudley White, was the perfect person to explain to the American public what had happened when he held a press conference three days later. The room was packed with reporters and television cameras. White, four years older than his patient, with his trim runner's frame, rimless glasses, and graying hair, spoke with a reassuringly genteel accent. He said that the president's heart attack was the result of one of his coronary arteries being blocked. White explained that the walls of these arteries tend to thicken as men reach middle age and become more likely to get blocked (due to what we now call atherosclerosis), and that this particular problem had become much more common in the past few decades. In fact, he said, this was now the most common serious illness affecting middle-aged American men, and they were having more heart attacks than men in any other country.

As to what causes this dangerous thickening of the walls of the arteries, White allowed that a man's heredity, body build, occupation, stress and strain, diet, smoking, and alcohol use might be involved, but cautioned that "nobody has yet made an adequate study of these various underlying factors." But there was one man who was already absolutely certain that he knew exactly what was causing the increase in heart disease in American men: Ancel Keys, a fifty-one-year-old professor of physiology at the University of Minnesota, was convinced that the only thing that really mattered was how much fat Americans were eating.

Ancel Keys Shouts, "Fat Is the Villain!"

It was three years earlier that Professor Keys found his answer to America's heart disease epidemic, while sitting with his wife at an outdoor restaurant in sunny Naples, Italy, looking out at the sparkling blue waters of the Mediterranean.

He was there because a physician from Naples had told him that the men who lived there did not have heart attacks, a claim Keys very much doubted. After all, back in Minnesota, one in every seven businessmen was dying from a heart attack before age sixty-five. But Keys had found that his colleague's claim was true: Heart attacks were quite rare in workingmen in Naples, and Italian men in general had only one-third as many fatal heart attacks as American men.

As he watched the Italian families around him digging enthusiastically into heaping plates of pasta covered with thick fragrant sauces of tomatoes and vegetables, he thought he understood why. Italians ate meat only once or twice a week and very little milk, cream, or butter. As a result, they were eating *half* as much fat as Americans and so, Keys thought, it must be this low-fat Italian diet that protected Italian men from heart disease. Keys paid little attention at the time to the many other ways the Italian diet was different from the American diet: fifty-five times more olive oil; twice as much bread, pasta, and fish; a third more fruit and vegetables; half as much sugar; and thirty-five times more wine. (Many years later, Keys would come to embrace some of the other elements of this "Mediterranean diet.")

Even before his visit to Naples, Keys was already inclined to blame fat for the rise in heart disease, because he had found that putting Minnesota businessmen on a very low-fat diet lowered the cholesterol in their blood. And since the fatty deposits that block coronary arteries and cause heart attacks have a lot of cholesterol in them, it seemed to make sense that lowering cholesterol in the blood ought to help prevent heart disease. But there were two troubling problems. While many men with heart attacks had high cholesterol levels in their blood, most did not. And if you asked men to report on exactly what they ate, there was little connection between their diets and their blood cholesterol levels. Some men eat lots of fat and have low cholesterol; some eat very little fat and have high cholesterol. Even the amount of cholesterol present in the foods people eat, like eggs, has very little effect on the amount in their blood.

But as he sat there in sunny Naples, Keys decided that none of this mattered. It was not what any single person ate that was important—it was what *everyone* ate, what all the people in a country ate. Italians must have less heart disease because they ate much less fat than Americans, so all he needed to do was to get Americans to eat less fat and the heart disease epidemic would melt away.

Soon after Keys returned to Minnesota, he wrote up his wonderful new idea that fat in the diet was the cause of the American heart disease epidemic. He showed that, in six different countries, the more fat there was in the diet, the more deaths there were from heart attacks. Unfortunately, he failed to mention that there were diet and heart disease figures for sixteen other countries that he had chosen to ignore. If he had included the figures from all of these countries, there would have been no relationship at all between dietary fat and deaths from heart disease, as other researchers soon pointed out. In fact, the three countries where men had the lowest death rates and highest life expectancy—Norway, Sweden, and Denmark—had just as much fat in their diets as the United States. But this and other inconvenient facts were consistently ignored by Keys and his followers. Today, we have data for 165 different countries, and these current worldwide statistics show that people in countries with more fat in the diet actually have fewer deaths from heart disease.

Keys thought that fat in the American diet also explained why heart disease in men had more than doubled from 1910 to 1950: because the percentage of calories from fat in our food supply had increased from 32 percent to 40 percent during that forty-year span. Fat calories in Italy were just 20 percent, and he was sure if we could just lower our percentage down to 30 percent, we would be much better off. And this is exactly how your "daily allowance" of fat on a food label is calculated today; it is 30 percent of the calories in a 2,000-calorie diet. Critics of Keys would point to an abundance of other evidence that showed that Americans had been eating a diet high in fat and animal fat long before the rise in heart disease. In fact, as later critics also pointed out, the small increase in fat in our diet that Keys blamed for the epidemic of heart disease was largely due to an increase in the same polyunsaturated vegetable oils Keys would later claim were beneficial.

There were other jarring facts. For example, neither Keys nor anyone else seemed to notice that there had been no epidemic of heart disease in women, even though they had been eating the same foods as men. In fact, deaths from heart disease in women had been slowly *declining* since the 1930s. Nor did anyone notice that something else had been increasing in American men at exactly the same time as heart disease: cigarette smoking, which, it turns out, triples the risk of a heart attack.

At the time of Eisenhower's heart attack, Keys had already been promoting his ideas about fat and heart disease for three years, but no one had paid much attention. But now suddenly everyone was interested. Three weeks after Ike's attack, *Time* magazine ran a cover story on heart disease in which Keys explained that the amount of fat in the American diet was the key to heart disease and that heredity, race, smoking, and obesity were much less important. A month later, *Reader's Digest* featured a long article on Keys's ideas about the evils of dietary fat: "Is This the No. 1 Villain in Heart Disease?"

Inspired by Keys's ideas, General Mills became the first food company to claim it had a product that could reduce the chances of heart disease because it was low in fat: "Wheaties may actually help you live longer! Recent studies indicate that common heart ailments are more prevalent in groups living on high fat diets." They all but quoted Keys: "We all need some fat. But *40 to 50 percent* of all calories in the average American diet are *fat*! Far too much, caution many nutrition authorities." Well, at least one authority. And so began Keys's epic collaboration with the food makers to instruct the American public about the evils of certain kinds of fat and the virtues of their products.

Unfortunately for Keys—and, as it turns out, for the rest of us—just when the press and the public were getting on board with his antifat campaign, new evidence turned up that not all fats were bad. While *saturated* fat, like the fat from meat and dairy foods, could raise the level of cholesterol in the blood, *polyunsaturated* fat, found mostly in vegetable oils like corn and soybean oil, did not. In fact, large amounts of corn oil could actually lower cholesterol.

The only way we can get these polyunsaturated fats is from what we eat, because our bodies cannot make them. They come in two forms: omega-3 and omega-6. Because corn oil is quite high in the omega-6 fat called *linoleic acid*, this was mistakenly given credit for lowering cholesterol when it was actually something else in the corn oil (sitosterol) that was responsible. But the belief that omega-6 linoleic is beneficial has persisted.

Keys was very slow to admit that different kinds of fat have different effects—even though he quickly confirmed this in his own laboratory—because it distracted people from his "fat is the villain" message. But a big and insatiable genie was out of the bottle as food industry executives smelled a new source of profits. For them, the idea that polyunsaturated fat was healthier could not have come at a better time. They were already using more vegetable oil—especially soybean oil—high in polyunsaturated fat in their food products because it was cheaper and easier to use than animal fat. And they also knew that because women want to give their families healthy foods, pitching their advertising in terms of health benefits would be a good way to sell them.

The Polyunsaturated Explosion

Quickly responding to the new research suggesting that polyunsaturated fats might be better than saturated fats, the Corn Products Refining Company debuted Mazola Corn Oil, promoting it as "unsaturated" and "nutritionally unexcelled." As the company's vice president modestly explained: "We don't want to appear to be medical men, but if Mazola can be used to alleviate nutritional malfunctions or improve anyone's health then obviously we're all for it—and no one can hurt himself by eating Mazola."

Despite the enthusiasm of the ad companies, most physicians remained skeptical about Keys's ideas. Joining with Keys in a telethon to raise money for the American Heart Association, Eisenhower's sainted cardiologist, Paul Dudley White, stunned his cohost by publically rejecting his diet-heart theory: "See here, I began my practice as a cardiologist in 1921 and I never saw an MI [heart attack] patient until 1928. Back in the MI-free days before 1920, the fats were butter and lard and I think that we would all benefit from the kind of diet that we had at a time when no one had ever heard the word corn oil." White knew that vegetable oils had been increasing in the American diet during the time when heart disease was going up. In fact, the share of calories from polyunsaturated fat had *doubled* from 1910 to the 1950s, while saturated fat had only increased by one-fifth.

The physician president of the American Heart Association now decided it was time for his public service group to weigh in on diet and heart disease. He asked four other expert physicians to join him in reviewing the evidence and invited Keys to present his ideas. Much to Keys's dismay, the panel's published report poked holes in every part of his argument. The panelists rejected his view that Americans were eating more fat than they used to, pointing to plenty of evidence of high fat intakes in the past, just as Dr. White had. Also, just as Keys himself had found, they noted that what people eat is not strongly related to the level of their blood cholesterol and that the cholesterol level is not a very good predictor of heart disease risk.

Worst of all, they rejected Keys's central argument that the number of heart disease deaths is strongly linked to the amount of fat in a country's diet, pointing to the many countries with high-fat diets and low heart disease rates. They also noted that countries with fewer deaths from heart disease often have more deaths from other causes and shorter overall life spans, something that Keys also found in his own studies. Yet for the next thirty years, diet-heart enthusiasts constantly referred to Keys's argument based on six or seven countries as the *strongest* and most convincing evidence for a link between diet and heart disease. They had to fall back on this, because there weren't any studies showing that changing your diet lowers your risk of heart disease.

Keys Strikes Back:
Eat Well and Stay Well (1959)

Because Keys was completely certain that the only way to reduce heart disease in American men was to get all Americans to change their diet, rejection by the American Heart Association was a serious setback. Since he couldn't win over the doctors, he decided to take his case directly to the people. So he and his wife, Margaret, wrote a book, *Eat Well and Stay Well*; and much to their delight, it became a best seller.

Here he proclaimed the goal that you can still find enshrined on every package of food you buy: "Keep total fats under 30% of your diet calories." Saturated fat is especially bad: "Restrict saturated fats, the fats in beef, pork, lamb, sausages, margarine, solid shortenings, fats in dairy products." Poultry escaped this censure; Keys thought that it was healthier because it has less saturated and more polyunsaturated fat than red meat. He also told his readers to "prefer vegetable oils to solid fats" and to favor the polyunsaturated fats that may reduce cholesterol, like corn oil and soybean oil. Keys rejected the idea that the trans fats created by hydrogenating soybean oil were unhealthy, because he had found that hydrogenated oil did not raise cholesterol levels in the blood. (Later it was found that trans fats dramatically lower high-density lipoprotein—HDL—the "good" cholesterol.)

Companies like Mazola and Wesson were paying close attention to Keys and quickly ramped up their health claims about the benefits of polyunsaturated oils and the evils of saturated fats. More and more ads appeared claiming that polyunsaturated fats in cooking oils, salad dressings, shortenings, and margarines could help to reduce cholesterol and prevent heart disease. Since there was little concrete evidence linking diet, cholesterol, and heart disease, officials at the U.S. Food and Drug Administration tried to stem this tide; but it did not matter—the deluge of ads continued. (Today anyone can make any health claim they want about any food, vitamin, or nutrient—as in the days of patent medicines—but until quite recently you were supposed to only make claims that were proven.)

After the success of his book, Keys was able to persuade the American Heart Association to change its mind and endorse his views by packing the medical committee with his supporters and persuading the vegetable oil makers to agree to support and fund the association. But the American Medical Association continued to strongly disagree, siding with the FDA's view that there was no proof of a link between diet and heart disease. A few years later the American Heart Association, flush with contributions from vegetable oil makers, recommended that *all* Americans should reduce fat in their diets and substitute polyunsaturated vegetable fat for saturated animal fats, even though it acknowledged that there was no actual proof that this would be beneficial. Since so many Americans are dying of heart attacks, the association said, we cannot wait for proof. The FDA found that most Americans already believed that polyunsaturated fats could prevent heart disease despite the lack of any evidence—as they still do. Because of this lack of evidence, the FDA tried again in vain to rein in the food makers but to no avail. The barrage of ads promoting "healthy" polyunsaturated in place of saturated fats continued unabated.

Keys's Victory Is Complete:
The 1977 *Dietary Goals for the United States*

As if the public needed any more convincing, in 1977, the staff of George McGovern's Senate Special Committee for Nutrition and Human Needs decided it was time for the government to tell Americans just what they should be eating in order to reduce coronary disease and other "killer diseases." Based entirely on the work of Keys and his disciples, the *Dietary Goals* put together by the Senate committee sanctified his ideas and will be quite familiar to anyone who has looked at a food label. They were exactly what Keys had been pushing for throughout the previous twenty years: We should reduce total fat to 30 percent of calories and saturated fat to 10 percent while *increasing* polyunsaturated fat by two-thirds, from 6 percent to 10 percent. Although the document did not say so explicitly, meeting these three fat goals would also require a 40 percent reduction in monounsaturated fat, the kind of fat found in olive oil and now considered beneficial.

In addition, we were told to cut sugar calories by half and double our starches to form the base of the new "food pyramid." To meet these goals, we should eat less red meat and eggs, avoid dairy fat, increase poultry and fish, and use more polyunsaturated oils high in omega-6 linoleic acid, like corn oil and hydrogenated soybean oil, just as Keys had said in his book two decades earlier.

The *Dietary Goals* unleashed a firestorm of criticism from the medical community, and at new hearings, the doctors in charge of the American Medical Association and the government's own National Heart, Lung, and Blood Institute both testified that there was no medical evidence to support the *Dietary Goals*. Many other expert physicians also opposed the recommendations. George Mann, the doctor who had first discovered that corn oil lowers cholesterol, testified against the recommendations and also warned about the high levels of unnatural trans fats in hydrogenated vegetable oils, a warning that went unheeded for twenty years. Despite all of these objections, the *Dietary Goals* were printed again at the end of the year (with a few changes to mollify the meat industry) and have been reissued every five years as *Dietary Guidelines for Americans* with few changes ever since. A 2010 review of the current *Dietary Guidelines* notes that the same criticisms leveled against the original version still apply today, because there is still no good evidence supporting their recommendations.

Game Over

By 1983, five years after the *Dietary Goals* were issued, surveys showed that most Americans believed that cholesterol causes coronary heart disease and can be lowered by cutting down on saturated fat and increasing polyunsaturated fat, just as the ads had been telling them. In contrast, given the lack of good scientific evidence, most physicians still did not accept the connection between dietary fat, cholesterol, and heart disease. Convincing the public through advertising had been much more successful than convincing the doctors (a lesson that was not lost on drug companies). The last great effort to prove that changing the diet can decrease heart disease, the MRFIT study, had failed to show any benefit, and many other studies had produced similar negative results. In fact, no large-scale study has ever shown that changing fat in the diet in accordance with the *Dietary Goals* lowers the death rate or extends life.

Physicians at the government's National Heart, Lung, and Blood Institute gave up on trying to show that changing the diet could lower cholesterol or reduce deaths from heart disease, and instead focused all of their efforts on trying to find drugs that would lower cholesterol in the blood. One trial after another had to be stopped because the drugs were causing excessive numbers of deaths, but researchers finally found a drug (cholestyramine) that lowered cholesterol by a small amount and had a very small *nonsignificant* effect in decreasing heart disease deaths and no effect at all on total deaths.

This very marginal result led to an immediate declaration of victory and the convening of a "consensus conference" by the National Heart, Lung, and Blood Institute whose outcome was predetermined before it started. Since lowering the cholesterol in the blood with cholestyramine was claimed to have a very small beneficial effect, the panel decided that changing to the diet advocated by Keys would also be helpful, though no studies had shown this. Despite the testimony of a number of leading researchers in the field strongly opposing any recommendation to change the American diet, the handpicked panel endorsed the creation of a National Cholesterol Education Program built around a strict Keys-type diet for virtually all Americans and the labeling of all foods for their fat content. Although there was still no evidence that changing your diet would lower your risk of heart disease, the panel went along with this because the members believed that the kind of diet advocated by Keys was probably not harmful, might help to *reduce* obesity (a very unfortunate mistake), and was not worth fighting since Keys's views were already accepted by the public.

Nothing had really changed since the American Heart Association had rejected Keys's views in 1957. There was still no evidence that increased fat in the diet had caused the coronary heart disease epidemic in American men. Changing the diet had little effect on cholesterol in the blood. And there was no convincing evidence that reducing fat and saturated fat or increasing polyunsaturated fat in the diet could prevent heart disease deaths and increase life span.

The campaign to get American women to change their families' diets waged over the past forty years was not based on sound science. It was consistently opposed by many physicians, including most of those who had done key research on diet and heart disease. Once launched by Keys, it was driven by aggressive advertising by the edible-oils and processed-food industries, marketing that consistently exaggerated and misrepresented the science and overwhelmed the feeble efforts of the FDA to limit overblown claims.

Keys himself later backed away from the monster he had helped to create. In an interview in 1987, he said, "I've come to think that cholesterol is not as important as we used to think it was. Let's reduce it by reasonable means, but let's not get too excited about it." In fact, Keys's own research failed to show any relationship between polyunsaturated fat in the diet and death rates.

So now that you know why the American diet changed, it's time to turn to the sad story of how those changes, intended to make us healthier, ended up making us fat instead.

CHAPTER 2

"No Good Deed Goes Unpunished": Why We Got Fatter

Sometimes, as she lies in bed in the morning, Susan remembers waking up as a child on her grandparents' farm to the smell of fresh-baked bread and coffee cake in the oven and the seductive tang of frying bacon mingled with a rich undercurrent of fresh ground coffee. And what a wonderful breakfast it was, with everyone sitting around the table eyeing the food with delight and digging in with gusto! Two or three eggs fried in bacon grease, thick slices of bacon, sausage, or ham, one or two tall frosty glasses of unashamedly full-fat milk, great slabs of bread made with bacon grease shortening and a butter crust and slathered in still more butter, coffee cake or pancakes also made with bacon grease, and cereal covered in delicious sweet cream. As good as the food tasted, somehow it was more satisfying as well. Everyone ate until they were full and went on with their work until it was time for the next meal. *And no one was fat.*

Where did all that wonderful food go? she wonders. And if it was so bad for us, why did the farmers live so much longer than city people? If only food still tasted as good as it did back then, before all the changes were made to make it "healthier." Well, what can you do? It's time for her to get up and have her usual morning meal, a bowl of granola with soy milk.

Meanwhile, four thousand miles away in Copenhagen, Denmark, forty-five-year-old Ingrid is sitting down to a breakfast very much like the one Susan used to have when she was a child. Back then, the Danish and American diets were a lot alike, with about a quarter of the calories coming from animal fat and a fifth from sugar. The weights of women in the two countries were also similarly low, and Danish men were among the healthiest in Europe. Today the Danish diet is still much as it used to be, with an even higher share of the calories coming from animal fat, plenty of sugar, and only one-fifth as many calories from vegetable oils as the American diet, and less than a tenth as much soybean oil. Ingrid, typical of Danish women in their forties, is an inch taller than Susan and weighs 145 pounds, just what American women used to weigh. Only one Danish woman in fourteen is obese compared with one in three American women. And the death rate from coronary disease in Denmark is 25 percent lower than in the United States even though the Danes spend less than half as much on health care as we do. Is it possible that the changes we Americans made in our diets might help to explain why Susan weighs so much more than Ingrid?

Some claim that our current American diet is filled with foods that taste so good we cannot control how much we eat. But for those like Susan who can still remember a time when animal fats were an unashamedly major part of our diet, as they still are for Europeans, food has never tasted as good as it did then. Even lovers of today's junk food would be quite surprised by how much better a Hostess cupcake or Twinkie or potato chip or french fry tasted when it was made with animal fat, and how much more satisfying it was.

Did we actually voluntarily give up most of these delicious foods in the quest to make ourselves healthier? Amazingly, we did. American women made unpleasant, unappealing, and difficult changes in the foods their families ate, and especially the fats they were eating, because they believed that this would improve their health. Instead we all got fatter. Here is a paradox: As the American diet has changed to make it "healthier," food got less tasty, and yet Americans—especially women—started gaining weight.

In fact, our weight began to increase at exactly the same time we began making changes in our national diet, the very changes advocated by Keys and the *Dietary Goals*. That both weight and diet changed at the same time suggests that those changes might be connected. And it seems reasonable to think that there must be some connection between our diet and our rising weight. But what could the connection be? Since fat has more than twice as many calories as sugar, it is an obvious suspect; but sugar is always on the list of possible evildoers and has certainly been accused by many of being responsible. And recently carbohydrates in general have been blamed. So let's start with them.

Could It Be Sugar or Carbohydrates?

Like many things we enjoy, sugar has a bad reputation. The nutritionists who wrote the *Dietary Goals* wanted us to cut the amount we eat by *half*. So it is not surprising that sugar has been accused of being responsible for our recent weight gains, as in David Kessler's bestselling book, *The End of Overeating*. Kessler believes that most of us are addicted to sugar (and fat) and that when sugar is added to processed foods, we cannot help eating more than we should. But if sugar were fueling our recent weight gains, we would expect its share of our calories to have gone up; instead, it's actually now a *smaller* share than it was in 1961. So it's difficult to see how it can be the culprit. We do eat 50 percent more sugar than the average European; but back in 1961, when our weights were similar to theirs, we ate even more—almost twice as much as they did. And today we eat about the same amount as the willowy Danes.

Do heavier American women eat more sugar? No. If we divide a large group of adult American women into a heavier half and a lighter half, we can compare their detailed reports of what they eat in a typical day. These dietary reports show that the lighter women actually have *more* sugar calories in their diets than the heavier women. Despite the almost universal condemnation of sugar by nutritionists, most other studies also show that heavier women do not eat more sugar, while lighter women often do.

But wait. While the total amount of sugars in our diet has not gone up, the *source* of our sugar has changed dramatically. We now eat only about half as much of the white granulated sugar that comes from sugar cane or sugar beets, having replaced much of it with "high-fructose corn syrup" added to processed foods. Processed-food makers prefer corn syrup because the vast river of government-subsidized corn flowing out of America's heartland has made it very cheap. And because corn syrup use has been increasing at the same time that our weights have gone up, it makes a plausible suspect.

But it turns out that granulated sugar and corn syrup sugar are really quite similar. Granulated sugar is an equal mixture of two simple sugars, glucose and fructose. Fructose gets its name from being common in fruit. Corn sugar is also a mixture of glucose and fructose, and despite its name, high-fructose corn syrup is not very high in fructose. Some types actually have *less* fructose than cane sugar and some have a bit more, but all are still more than two-fifths glucose. So there is no reason to think that corn syrup would have a much different effect on our bodies than cane sugar, and studies have not found that it does. Some studies do suggest that children who drink more sugary beverages weigh more than those who don't, but when sodas were sweetened with cane sugar instead of corn syrup a few decades ago, they had just as many calories and tasted just as sweet. If these beverages are contributing to recent weight gains, it's likely to be how much we're consuming rather than the source of the sugars they contain.

Sugars plus starches make up the carbohydrates, and recently the journalist Gary Taubes has popularized the idea that the carbs in our diet are the cause of our excess weight and that we should eliminate most of those and eat more meat. But women's weights are higher in countries where there is more meat in the diet and lower where there are more carbs. In addition, back in 1910, when Americans were much thinner, carbs made up a significantly *greater* share of our calories than they do now, while the share from meat was the same. And finally, American women also tend to weigh less when they eat more carbs and weigh more when they eat more meat. So it is hard to see how sugar or carbs can be to blame.

What About Fat?

Because of its bounty of calories—more than twice as many as the same amount of sugar—it is quite tempting to blame fat for our woes. It seems natural to think that eating more fat should make us fatter. One reason that some physicians reluctantly went along with the Keys diet was that cutting fat was supposed to make us thinner. David Kessler claims that the fat added to processed foods (along with the sugar) also makes us want to eat more and so leads us to gain weight. But during the time when our weights were going up, we were doing our best to follow Keys's advice to eat less fat, not more.

When asked to give their families "healthier" food, American women tried to do the right thing and choose foods with less fat. As you might expect with all of the "low-fat" products lining our grocery store shelves, the calorie share of fat in our diets did go down. From the late 1960s to the late 1990s, fat calories fell from 42 percent to 36 percent, and the share from monounsaturated fat decreased by a tenth. But then the fat percentage started heading back up to 41 percent as many of us tried to stem the tide of rising weight with one of the then-popular low-carb, high-fat diets.

So what actually happened when we were eating less fat? During the thirty years that the calorie share of fat in our diets was going down, our weights were going sharply up. And when we look at other evidence, there is little to suggest that fat intake is related to weight. In Europe, where women typically weigh twenty pounds less than we do, their calorie share from fat is just 4 percent less than ours. And the food reports from thousands of American women do not show that those who eat more fat weigh more. So it is hard to blame the total amount of fat in our diets for our weight gain. Could it be some particular kind of fat that is to blame?

Saturated Fat

Because Keys and his disciples told us that saturated fat is supposed to be especially bad for us, Americans have tried hard to eat less of it. In fact, we had better success with this goal than with decreasing fat overall. In the two decades following the publication of the *Dietary Goals* we did especially well. By the late 1990s we had cut saturated fat from 16 percent of our calories down to 11 percent, though it has since crept back up to 13 percent (just where it was in 1910). We also changed where our saturated fat was coming from. In 1910, before anyone knew what a heart attack was, most of our fat came from animals and 90 percent of our saturated fat came from meat, eggs, and dairy foods. Today, the majority of our saturated fat comes from the refined vegetable oils added to our food by processed-food makers. And while Europeans have about the same amount of saturated fat in their diets as we do, much more of theirs is still animal fat. They eat almost twice as much lard and butter as we do, adding up to a full 8 percent of their calories. Since Europeans weigh much less than we do, this kind of saturated fat must not be very fattening. And American women who eat more saturated fat are no heavier than those who eat less of it.

But is it possible that the story runs the other way: that eating *less* of these saturated animal fats could be linked to our recent weight gains? One hundred years ago, when most of our fat came from animals and almost half was saturated, the average weight for an American woman in her late forties was 145 pounds. In the 1960s, when Americans' calorie share of saturated fat was a little larger, women's weights were about the same. We also know from studying their bones that our Stone Age ancestors had a diet with plenty of meat and animal fat. Likewise, people who still live like our ancient ancestors, hunting and gathering their foods, also have diets with a substantial amount of meat and saturated animal fat. So this seems to be the kind of diet we evolved to eat. In addition, for the past five thousand years, many of us have supplemented fat from meat with dairy fat, which is also high in saturated fat, though Americans have cut back on many dairy foods during the last forty years, the same period when we were gaining weight.

Here, the story may be the reverse of popular belief: Having less dairy fat could be a factor in our rising weight. In 1961, dairy foods accounted for more than a sixth of our calories; today, they add up to less than a tenth. Europeans consume much more dairy foods than we do, especially butter and cheese, particularly the slender French. Lighter American women also tend to eat more dairy foods, drink more milk, and have more yogurt and natural cheese than heavier women. Many studies also support the idea that having more dairy food is linked to lower weights. Most dairy products have added vitamin D, which is also linked to lower weights. The more vitamin D American women have in their blood, the lower their weights tend to be, and our vitamin D levels have been falling as we have been gaining weight. So our cutting back on dairy foods could have also played some part in our weight gain.

The Oiling of Americans

Now it's time to turn our attention to the eight-hundred-pound gorilla in the room. When it comes to the dietary goal of increasing polyunsaturated fat and omega-6 linoleic acid—the kind in purified vegetable oils—we have done an outstanding job. The single biggest change in the American diet over the past forty years has been an enormous increase in vegetable oils high in polyunsaturated fat. We have almost doubled their share of the calories in our diet—from one-ninth to one-fifth of all of our calories. In the American food supply, there are now six and a half gallons of vegetable oil a year for each man, woman, and child, almost a third of a cup a day. More than three-quarters of this vegetable oil is soybean oil (five hundred calories a day), which is seven times more soybean oil than in the European diet and much more than *any other country in the world.* Most of the rest of our vegetable oil is corn oil, and we eat five times more of this than the Europeans. Our voracious appetite for soybean and corn oil is the biggest difference between our diet today and the diet of the much thinner Europeans or the diet we used to have before we started gaining weight.

More than half of the vegetable oil we consume is polyunsaturated fat, mostly omega-6 linoleic acid, the same kind of fat that was mistakenly believed to lower our cholesterol. The amount of polyunsaturated omega-6 fat in our diet has more than doubled and now supplies more than *10 percent* of all our calories. We do need some omega-6, but a diet this high in omega-6 linoleic is unprecedented in human existence and extremely unnatural. It would be impossible to consume this much omega-6 without the heavy industrial processing of corn and soybeans. Most vegetables are low in fat, with no more than 1 or 2 percent. Because extracting and purifying corn or soybean oil is a complex chemical process, before the past century vegetable oils were never a significant part of our diets.

In the Stone Age diet, as many as three-fifths of all calories came from fat, but most of this fat came from animals and was saturated or monounsaturated (like the fat in olive oil). In grass-fed beef, for example, half of the fat is saturated and most of the rest is monounsaturated. Less than 5 percent is polyunsaturated fat, and much of that is the beneficial omega-3 type rather than the omega-6 found in vegetable oils. In 1910, when most of the fat in our diets still came from animals, less than a tenth of our fat was polyunsaturated, supplying less than 3 percent of our calories. So there was very little polyunsaturated fat in our diets at a time when coronary disease was virtually unknown, just as Paul Dudley White pointed out to Ancel Keys many years ago. In fact, as we have seen, the amount of polyunsaturated vegetable fat in our diets started to go up at the same time that heart disease was increasing.

The purified corn and soybean oils that now supply so many of our calories bear little relationship to the foods that they come from. Corn itself is less than 2 percent oil while soybeans are 7 percent. Both have substantial amounts of protein, starch, sugars, and a variety of minerals and vitamins, just as foods usually do. But in the processed purified oils, virtually all of these nutrients are gone. Only a few vitamins, ones that dissolve in fat, like vitamin E, remain. Without using tons of industrial chemicals, these oils would be inedible. They are not foods;

they are artificial chemical products—"food-like substances" as the journalist and food advocate Michael Pollan would say.

From the viewpoint of Keys and his disciples, the enormous increase in polyunsaturated oils and omega-6 linoleic acid in the American diet should have been very beneficial. It was just what they were hoping for. The *Dietary Goals* wanted us to increase polyunsaturates from 6 percent to 10 percent of our calories, and especially increase omega-6 linoleic, the kind of fat that was supposed to lower cholesterol. Unfortunately, this is just what we did. To help us choose vegetable oils high in linoleic, the *Dietary Goals* included a list of oils showing the amount of linoleic in each. Because they are both quite high in linoleic, *hydrogenated* soybean oil and corn oil were near the top of this list, and Keys also listed these as desirable vegetable oils in his book. So increasing polyunsaturated vegetable oils high in omega-6 linoleic is exactly what was supposed to help lower our blood cholesterol level. Unfortunately, as we now know, both corn and soybean oil lower our *good* cholesterol, or HDL; and to make matters even worse, until quite recently, nearly all of the soybean oil in our diets has been *hydrogenated*, creating harmful trans fats, which actually *increase* the risk of heart disease and may also increase the risk of certain cancers.

Why Soybean Oil and Corn Oil Increased

It would be nice to report that food makers put more polyunsaturated vegetable oil into our foods because they thought this would make us healthier. After all, Keys and his supporters thought that increasing these oils should be beneficial, and the vegetable oil companies did pay for some research attempting to document health benefits. In turn, those alleged health benefits certainly made it easier for food makers to promote processed-food products with added vegetable oils as healthy, and for women to accept them as desirable when these polyunsaturated oils were used in place of supposedly harmful saturated fats.

But the goal for Americans to increase polyunsaturated fat seems to have been a marvelous and unexpected gift for the food makers that they did their best to exploit. The real reason they were using more soybean and corn oil was that—when chemically processed—these oils were much cheaper than animal fats and more stable and easy to use. Because of these economic advantages, vegetable oils and polyunsaturated fats had been slowly increasing in our diet since the 1940s, long before anyone started thinking of them as healthy. As we have seen, this was one of the things that Keys's critics found especially irritating: The small increase in fat in the American diet that he blamed for the epidemic of heart disease was mostly due to an increase in the very same polyunsaturated vegetable oils he claimed were good for us!

American farmers began planting more soybeans in the 1930s with financial help from the federal government in order to add back nitrogen to the depleted soil in the "dust bowl" of the American heartland. It was a pleasant surprise when soybeans turned out to be a very valuable crop. Most of them are crushed to squeeze out the oil, and a variety of industrial chemicals are then used to degum, refine, bleach, and deodorize the oil, which is otherwise inedible. The solid part of the soybean that is left behind is used to add protein to feeds for chickens, cows, and pigs.

But regular soybean oil has one very serious drawback for food makers. Almost 7 percent of the oil is the *omega-3* fatty acid called *alpha-linolenic*, the most basic and most common form of omega-3 fat. And while omega-3 fats are very beneficial for our weight and health, they are a disaster for food makers. Because all omega-3s, including alpha-linolenic, are very active chemically, they tend to react with oxygen in the air and become rancid and taste and smell bad over time, which is not a quality food makers want. But there is a way around this. Exposing the oil to a carefully controlled amount of hydrogen gas can convert the omega-3 alpha-linolenic into omega-6 linoleic. This also improves the flavor of the oil, lightens the color, and helps to keep it from turning rancid because omega-6 fats are much less reactive than omega-3. For this reason, until quite recently, almost all soybean oil was at least *"partially hydrogenated"* in this way. Anyone who has read the ingredients on a food label will have often seen "partially hydrogenated soybean oil." Adding even more hydrogens to the oil converts some of the monounsaturated to saturated fat, making it solid enough to be suitable for shortening or margarine.

Unfortunately, artificially adding hydrogens to a fatty acid twists the chemical bond and turns it into an unnatural trans fat. As many as half of the fatty acids in hydrogenated soybean oil are converted to trans fats. But even though most soybean oil and much of the corn oil in our diets was hydrogenated, Keys and his followers did not see this as a problem because they had found that trans fats did not raise cholesterol levels in the blood. No one seemed to notice that they took away much of the HDL, the *good* cholesterol. And unnatural trans fats were also a boon for processed-food makers because they make food even more resistant to spoiling and turning rancid.

By the end of the twentieth century, nearly all of the fat in American processed food was coming from soybean oil, with most of it either partially hydrogenated to produce cooking and salad oils or more heavily treated with hydrogen to make shortening and margarine. We now know that this was not good for us. Although vegetable oils were supposed to lower our risk of heart disease, trans fats increase that risk more than any other kind of food, and even small amounts of trans fats have a measureable harmful effect. Unfortunately, just as in the case of tobacco, evidence that trans fats were harmful was intentionally suppressed for many years. After trans fats were finally acknowledged to be unhealthy, seed companies quickly developed a new breed of soybeans with very low levels of omega-3, and this is now the type planted by many farmers. Even without trans fats, the oil made from this new type of low-omega-3 soybeans is even higher in the obesity-promoting omega-6 and lower in health-promoting omega-3.

So where is all of this soybean and corn oil in our food? Maybe we use a little vegetable oil when we cook and in our salad dressings, but this surely doesn't come to a third of a cup a day. The answer is that most of it is hidden in our food in the form of commercial cooking oils and vegetable shortenings added to processed foods. In 1960, these made up less than a fifth of all the fat in our diet; today they are *half*! At the same time that food makers have been switching from animal fats to vegetable oils in their products, we have been getting more and more of our diet from these prepared or processed foods. Today, there are thirty-two pounds of cooking oil and twenty-two pounds of shortening in foods for each American a year compared with just four pounds each of butter and margarine and two pounds of salad dressing.

Much of the thirty-two pounds of cooking oil is used for frying. A single potato chip, for example, is two-fifths vegetable oil and has nearly a gram of fat. A typical french fry or onion ring is also one-fifth oil, with more than a gram of fat. While a plain roasted chicken wing is already 8 percent fat, transformed into a buffalo wing it is more than a fifth fat, with more than five grams. Even "butter-flavored" popcorn is one-third vegetable oil.

The other hidden fat in our food is the twenty-two pounds of vegetable shortening. To make tasty well-textured baked goods—most breads and virtually all pastries, pie crusts, cookies, cakes, muffins—you need "shortening" to break up the gluten strands in the flour and make the dough finer, flakier, and more flavorful. This shortening used to be animal fat, like butter, lard, or bacon grease; but in 1911, Procter & Gamble first introduced Crisco, a shortening made by hydrogenating vegetable oil. It was snow-white, bland, and odorless, and, unlike lard, it could be kept at room temperature for long periods of time. Today, more than a fourth of the omega-6 linoleic in our diet comes from vegetable oil shortening in baked goods.

Omega-6 in Vegetable Oils Makes Us Fatter

Unfortunately, it appears that the enormous and unnatural increase in industrially produced soybean and corn oils in the American diet is what has made us fatter. In 165 countries around the world, women weigh more where there is more corn and soybean oil in the diet. With seven times more soybean oil and five times more corn oil in her diet, the average American woman weighs twenty pounds more than the average European.

The main reason that soybean and corn oils promote weight gain is because of the very large amounts of polyunsaturated omega-6 *linoleic acid* that they contain, the very oil that was supposed to lower our cholesterol but doesn't. More than half of the fat in soybean and corn oil is linoleic. As a result, today in the American food supply, there are twelve teaspoons of linoleic a day for each of us, far more than for any other country, accounting for more than 10 percent of all our calories. There is no way we could be getting this much omega-6 linoleic without purifying vegetable oils with industrial chemicals. But what does omega-6 fat have to do with our weight?

In the late 1990s, researchers in Heidelberg, Germany, enrolled eleven thousand women aged thirty-five and older in a six-year study of dietary fat and weight gain. At the beginning of the study, the average woman weighed 149 pounds with a BMI of 25; and she gained two pounds over the six years, though some gained much more. Why did some women gain more and some less? The researchers found that *the single dietary factor most strongly related to women's weight gain was the amount of omega-6 linoleic acid in their diet.* And the definition of "high" linoleic intake they used in the study was *25 percent lower* than the *average* intake for American women. Women were also more likely to gain more weight when they had more *arachidonic acid* in their diets, the active form of omega-6, which we can either make from linoleic or get from our diet. Women who ate more of either of these two forms of omega-6, linoleic and arachidonic, were especially likely to gain more than ten pounds.

Omega-6 linoleic itself does not seem to have any function in our bodies, but we convert it into arachidonic, the most important and potent form of omega-6 and a powerful promoter of weight gain. The more linoleic acid in our diets, the more arachidonic we make. In addition to having very large amounts of omega-6 linoleic, the American diet also has much higher levels of preformed arachidonic than the diet in most other countries. As the German study showed, higher levels of omega-6 linoleic and arachidonic in the diet are both strongly related to women's weights when we compare different countries or American women with different weights. In addition, many studies show that obese adults and children have higher levels of linoleic and arachidonic in their blood, all of which come from the omega-6 in their diets. Giving lab animals more linoleic acid, arachidonic acid, or soybean oil also makes them gain weight. We Americans get much more of these omega-6 fats that increase weight than anyone else: more arachidonic and more of the omega-6 linoleic, which converts to arachidonic in our bodies.

So how much does the exceedingly high level of omega-6 in the American diet relate to women's weights? As we might expect, heavier women report eating more high-omega-6 foods. However, we have found an even better way to see how strongly corn and soybean oil affect American women's weights. It turns out, quite by chance, that both oils happen to contain a large amount of a particular form of vitamin E—called *gamma-tocopherol*—which is rare in other foods. This means that the level of gamma-tocopherol in a woman's blood is a very good indicator of how much corn and soybean oil she is eating, and this level has been measured in thousands of American women along with other vitamins.

We find that the more gamma-tocopherol in the blood of American women, the more they weigh. This is one of our biggest discoveries. *Of all the factors that might be related to a woman's weight, the amount of gamma-tocopherol in her blood is the single best predictor of how much any particular American woman weighs.* Women under age fifty with very low levels of gamma-tocopherol in their blood weigh an average of 135 pounds compared to 220 pounds for those with the highest gamma-tocopherol levels. Since our bodies cannot make this vitamin, all of it comes from the diet; a woman's weight cannot change her gamma-tocopherol level. So it must be the foods that have a lot of gamma-tocopherol—corn and soybean oil—that are pushing up our weights. In addition, the women with more gamma-tocopherol also have much lower levels of HDL, the "good cholesterol," and other studies have also found that soybean oil lowers HDL.

Soybean and corn oil—and the high levels of omega-6 they

contain—may not only be making American women fatter, they may also be putting more of women's fat into their waists. Several studies have linked both trans fats and high omega-6 levels with larger waist sizes as well as higher weights. Waists normally expand as we gain weight, but the waist sizes of American women today are larger than we would expect for their weights and heights when compared with women twenty years ago. This increase in waist size has been even more dramatic in younger women, and this is probably because this age group has been exposed to a high-omega-6 diet for a larger fraction of their lives. Because of the staggering rise in vegetable oils in our diets, our waist fat is increasing even faster than our overall weight.

How Omega-6 Makes Us Fatter

The very high levels of omega-6 linoleic in our diet produce higher levels of arachidonic acid in our blood, and there is also more pre-formed arachidonic in our diets than in most other countries. But *how* does arachidonic affect our weight? One way it may make us heavier is by producing certain types of signaling molecules called eicosanoids. Eicosanoids made from arachidonic promote the growth and development of fatty tissue and fat storage. They also make our white blood cells more active and increase inflammation, which may contribute to blood vessel diseases in addition to promoting obesity. Omega-3 fats produce a different type of eicosanoid that has the opposite effects to those that come from omega-6; it decreases fat storage and opposes inflammation.

Perhaps even more significantly, omega-6 fats also make us fatter by increasing our body's own in-house version of marijuana. Just as our bodies make their own narcotics (called endorphins), they also make their own marijuana-like molecules out of arachidonic, the *endocannabinoids*. These natural fat molecules are quite similar to the active ingredient in marijuana. And just as marijuana is used medically to help stimulate the appetite of patients with cancer and AIDS, our own endocannabinoids also stimulate our appetites. Higher levels of endo-cannabinoids are found in obese people and in those with more waist fat, which could also help to explain why American waist sizes have been increasing. Since endocannabinoids are made from arachidonic, and arachidonic is made from linoleic, having such large amounts of omega-6 linoleic acid in our diet causes us to make much more appetite-stimulating endocannabinoid than usual.

In our quest to understand why Americans have been gaining so much extra weight, it seems that we have finally found a plausible suspect. It's not sugar, carbs, or fat in general that is making us heavy. Our weight increase is closely tied to the unprecedented amount of vegetable oil we are eating and the heavy doses of omega-6 fats those oils contain. And, as if that weren't bad enough, there is also another way that omega-6 makes us heavier.

Bad Fat Drives Away Good Fat

The other way the omega-6 in our diet makes us gain weight is by decreasing the good fat—omega-3—that makes us thinner. Just as linoleic is the most basic form of omega-6 fat, *alpha-linolenic acid* is at the root of the omega-3 family. Linoleic is like an evil twin, and alpha-linolenic, a good twin. We have seen that omega-6 linoleic is converted to arachidonic, which strongly promotes obesity. Using the very same process, omega-3 alpha-linolenic can be converted to EPA (eicosapentaenoic acid), and EPA, into DHA (docosahexaenoic acid)—the queen of omega-3 fats—which is especially important in the brain. EPA and DHA have exactly the opposite effect of arachidonic: They oppose weight gain. Where omega-6 increases weight, omega-3 lowers it. The more omega-3 a woman has in her diet, the lower her weight tends to be.

In the German study of dietary fat and weight gain, the *more* omega-3 fats in a woman's diet (alpha-linolenic, DHA, and EPA), the *less* weight she gained over time. Women's weights are lowest when they have more omega-3 *and* less omega-6 in their diet. For example, in Japan, where omega-3 DHA and EPA from the diet are very high and omega-6 quite low, very few women are obese—fewer than one in fifty! Many studies have shown that women and girls with more omega-3 and less omega-6 in their blood and diet weigh less. And several studies have shown that increasing omega-3 in the diet helps women to lose weight. Animals fed more omega-3 and less omega-6 also weigh less and are less likely to become obese. And omega-3 fat also has the opposite effect on the waist as omega-6, decreasing fat in the belly.

Omega-3 helps to reduce weight by increasing the burning of fat in the body and decreasing the amount of fat that we store. And where omega-6 increases appetite, omega-3 reduces it. People feel the hungriest after meals high in omega-6 linoleic and the least hungry after meals high in omega-3. Omega-3 fats also reduce the amount of insulin in our blood, the hormone that promotes fat storage.

Omega-6 and omega-3 fat groups are like two opposing families locked in a perpetual struggle for dominance. Whatever one does, the other does the opposite. Omega-6 increases weight, omega-3 lowers weight; omega-6 increases inflammation, omega-3 reduces it. We cannot make either one; they both have to come from our diet. But because these two omega groups compete with each other, when we add more omega-6 to our diet, it actively drives out the omega-3. Having more omega-6 in our diets pushes the omega-3 out of our bodies: When there is more omega-6 and linoleic in the diet and blood, there is less omega-3 in the blood.

One of the major battlefields in the struggle between omega-3 and omega-6 is over which family gets to make more of the active forms. In our bodies, omega-6 linoleic can be converted to arachidonic and omega-3 alpha-linolenic can be converted to EPA and then to DHA. Unfortunately, converting either omega-3 or omega-6 requires exactly the same chemical machinery, so the two types of omega fat constantly compete against each other for the right to use that machinery to move up to the next level. Whichever one has the most raw ingredients in the diet and blood, linoleic or alpha-linolenic, will be able to make more of the active forms, arachidonic or EPA and DHA.

The conversion process is like a lottery machine with both red and blue Ping-Pong balls bouncing around waiting for a chance to get sucked into the tube and onto the tray. If there are many more red balls than blue balls in the big container, many more red balls will naturally end up on the tray. In the same way, when there is much more omega-6 linoleic than omega-3 alpha-linolenic, as there now is in our diets, much more omega-6 arachidonic is made than omega-3 EPA and DHA. This means that there is much more of the omega-6 fat, which promotes weight gain (arachidonic), *as well as* less of the omega-3 fat, which reduces weight gain (EPA and DHA).

Plants usually have as much or more omega-3 than omega-6, so meat and eggs from the animals that eat them have a natural balance between omega-3 and omega-6. Our Stone Age ancestors probably had even more omega-3 than omega-6 from the foods they ate, which is the normal diet for our human species. But because of the staggering increase in vegetable oils in our diet, the balance between omega-6 and omega-3 has been reversed and become extremely lopsided. Fifty years ago there was already more omega-6 than omega-3 in our diet compared with the Stone Age diet. But since 1960, we have gone from having nine times more omega-6 than omega-3 to having more than *twenty-one times* as much. The omega-3 in our diets is now completely overwhelmed by the omega-6.

Making matters still worse, as our omega-6 has been zooming up, we have also been getting less omega-3 from some of the natural sources of omega-3 EPA and DHA in our diets: meat, poultry, eggs, and fish. The amount of omega fats in meat depends on what the animals eat; as Michael Pollan has memorably said, "You are what you eat eats." And most animals are now fed corn instead of grass because it's cheaper. Since corn is much higher in omega-6 and much lower in omega-3 than grass, this change in animal feeds has lowered the omega-3 in meat and eggs while increasing the omega-6. Naturally grass-fed animals have much more omega-3 and less omega-6 than those confined to sheds and barns. And while chicken meat and eggs still have some omega-3 EPA and DHA, they now have much more omega-6 than omega-3 because chickens have also been switched over to corn-based feed.

Fish and seafood are by far the best food sources of omega-3 because they have large amounts of active forms, EPA and DHA, but our high levels of omega-6 have also made it much harder for us to get that omega-3. To begin with, the share of fish in our diets has stayed about the same over the past forty years. Europeans eat *twice* as much fish as we do, and women weigh less in countries where people eat more fish. But we are also getting less omega-3 than we used to from the fish we do eat. One reason is that most farmed fish have more omega-6 and less omega-3 than wild-caught fish, especially farmed tilapia.

Even worse, when we eat any fish that is prepared or served with vegetable oils, as Americans usually do, we are unlikely to retain the valuable omega-3 present in the fish. Americans eat most of their fish fried and breaded or covered with batter, and studies have shown that when fish is eaten with vegetable oils in this way, the omega-3 it contains is no longer available to us. Heavier American women not only eat less fish than lighter women, they are much more likely to have their fish in combination with omega-6 vegetable oils. Their fish meals have almost *three times more omega-6* than the fish eaten by lighter women.

One way to see how the two competing kinds of omega fats in the diet affect women's weights is by looking at how much of each is in the breast milk of mothers in different countries and how that level relates to their weights. The fats in a mother's milk are the end result of all the competition between omega-6 and omega-3 in her body and show how much omega-3 has made it past the gauntlet of omega-6. We have collected data on the milk of mothers in over forty countries and recently teamed up with coworkers to analyze breast milk from an Amazonian tribe in Bolivia called the Tsimane. As expected, we find that women are very likely to weigh more when their breast milk has more omega-6 and less omega-3. As you would predict from their diet, American mothers have higher levels of omega-6 and much lower amounts of omega-3 in their breast milk than women in most other countries. In fact, the ratio of omega-6 (bad) to omega-3 (good) in our milk is almost twice as high as the *average* for the other countries where we have breast milk data. Sadly, this means that the amount of brain-building DHA in American mother's milk is also quite low, close to the lowest in the world and just half of the world average. Having more omega-6 *and* less omega-3 is especially likely to make our weights go up, and that's what American mothers are giving their babies from their very first meal.

So it now seems that shifting from animal fats to polyunsaturated vegetable oils was a really bad idea. It ended up bringing a lot of unnatural omega-6 and trans fats into our diet and pushing both the imbalance between omega-6 and omega-3 fats and our weights to unnaturally high levels. No one had any idea that our big diet and heart disease experiment would turn out this way.

Did Changing Our Diets Make Us Healthier or Sicker?

As we saw in the last chapter, there never was any compelling evidence to support the idea that changing the fat in our diets would make us healthier; but is it possible that it has made us *less* healthy? The increasing number of American men and women who are very obese has certainly not improved our nation's health. And the large amount of trans fats from hydrogenated oils in our diets cannot have been good for our hearts. The same is true of the doubling of the ratio of omega-6 to omega-3, since omega-6 fats promote inflammation while omega-3s oppose them and are strongly linked with lower rates of heart disease. It's also unlikely that we benefited by reducing our consumption of the health-promoting monounsaturated fats.

And while deaths from heart disease in Americans have been decreasing, as they have been all over the world, there are now sixty-two countries with lower heart disease rates than ours. Our rates are higher despite our spending *four times* as much money on health care as the average for those countries, giving a large percentage of our population cholesterol-lowering drugs, and performing millions of costly surgical procedures to ream out or replace blocked coronary arteries. And *every country* with a lower heart disease rate than ours has a higher level of omega-3 and lower amount of omega-6 in its diet than we do.

The main reason we were told to eat more polyunsaturated and less saturated fat was to lower the cholesterol in our blood. So did our new diet actually lower our cholesterol? Because most older men and women with high cholesterol levels have been treated with cholesterol-lowering drugs since the 1980s, this is not an easy question to answer. But most women in their thirties have not yet been prescribed these drugs, so we can look at whether the cholesterol levels have changed in this age group. The answer is no. The average cholesterol level for American women in their thirties is the same today as it was in the early 1970s.

So why did heart disease deaths go down? In American men, the death rate from heart disease peaked in 1963 and then began a sharp decline, well before any change in our diets. But that was the very same year when cigarette consumption by American males peaked and then began exactly the same decline. Cigarette consumption had gone up from less than one per week for each American male in 1900 to more than twenty per day by 1950, when the majority of American men were smoking, as accurately depicted in the television show *Mad Men.* As the number of cigarettes increased from year to year, deaths from heart disease in men went up. Then, when the number of cigarettes per male started to go steadily down in 1964, so did deaths from heart disease in men. Deaths from heart disease in men both rose and fell in exactly the same way as cigarette smoking, with smoking accounting for more than *90 percent* of the changes. Men who smoke are two to three times more likely to die from coronary heart disease; and from 1900 to 1963, the heart disease death rate in men increased by two and a half times, just what we would expect if smoking were the cause.

Because very few women smoked during the time that heart disease deaths were increasing in men, heart disease deaths did not increase in women; in fact, they gradually declined. But while women's smoking rates were much lower than men's, they went up in the 1960s and '70s, peaked in the early 1980s, and have since declined more slowly then men's. And while women's death rates from heart disease are much lower than men's, they have also been declining more slowly since the 1980s.

Because heart disease rates were already falling at the time when we began to decrease the amount of fat and saturated fat in our diets and increase polyunsaturated fat, the diet-heart enthusiasts were quite eager to take credit for the decline. But as heart disease deaths continued to fall at the same rate after Americans again increased their intake of "bad" fats, their enthusiasm was strangely muted.

The Final Verdict

To see the effect of the changes in our diet on our weight we have examined four separate lines of evidence—dietary changes in America over time, diet and weight differences between America and other countries, dietary differences between heavier and lighter American women, and the results of many medical studies that show how dietary factors affect weight. And they all agree on the most likely culprit driving weight gain in American women over the past forty years. Sugar and carbohydrates look to be innocent. On the other hand, the "good and healthy" fat of the *Dietary Goals*—omega-6 linoleic—is the prime suspect. High levels of omega-6 fat in our diets combined with low levels of omega-3 fat are strongly linked with both weight gain and increasing waist sizes, and American weights went up at exactly the same time that omega-6 increased in our diets. By trying to comply with misguided and baseless recommendations to change our diets, American women quite unintentionally made themselves and their families heavier. Their good deeds have been quite spectacularly punished. Or as Pogo used to say: We have met the enemy and he is us.

Part Two

Why Women Need Fat

CHAPTER 3

Why Women Have Curvy Hips

At age fifty-two, Professor Devendra Singh felt that his life was falling apart. The recession of 1990 had torpedoed his carefully developed real estate portfolio, forcing him into bankruptcy. His wife had filed for divorce. And he was lying in a hospital bed recovering from his third heart attack: not a very promising health record. Although Dev, as his colleagues called him, was admired as an inspiring teacher in the Psychology Department at the University of Texas, he had not published any new research in a while.

It had not been easy for Dev to become a psychology professor in the first place. Growing up in northern India, he defied his father to study philosophy and then psychology at Agra University. Again disobeying his father, he secretly left home in the middle of the night so that he could come to the United States and further his studies at Ohio State University. There he earned a doctorate in experimental psychology and moved on to a faculty position in Austin.

But now, Dev's world had narrowed down to the beeping of his heart monitor and the few people who entered his hospital room or passed by in the corridor; his active mind struggled against the tedium. Most of his visitors were attentive young nurses in trim white uniforms, and this got his psychologically trained mind wondering about what makes a woman attractive to men. He knew that social scientists generally believed that each culture has its own ideas about what is considered attractive and that fashions come and go, but he wondered whether there might be a deeper connection between a woman's body shape and her health. If there were, that might explain *why* certain shapes are attractive. So the next time his doctor came by, Dev asked him. And, sure enough, there was a connection.

One striking feature that makes a woman's body different from a man's is that her waist tends to be much smaller than her hips. And a number of medical studies had shown that women with larger waists and smaller hips—a higher "waist-hip ratio"—tended to have poorer health and were more likely to get diabetes and heart disease. So the shape of a woman's body *was* a clue to her health.

This insight would be the start of a dynamic new phase in Professor Singh's research career. His key idea was that attractiveness might not be simply a matter of fashion but, instead, something built into the brain. Most of his colleagues believed that people simply absorb their culture's traditions and beliefs about what is beautiful. They pointed to constant changes in fashions in how women look and dress and to the more extreme examples in groups where women made their necks longer with metal rings or put large plates in their lower lips to make themselves more attractive. Although the idea that all of our mental furniture comes from our culture is now slowly being abandoned by social scientists, Dev was among the first to question it. He thought that beauty might literally reside in the mind of the beholder, that attractiveness might be carrying some deeper message.

There was already evidence trickling in showing that similar ideas about attractiveness turn up in many different cultures. Working with many collaborators, David Buss, an American psychologist, had recently looked at what men and women in thirty-seven different cultural groups around the world thought was attractive and found that there was always the same big difference between the sexes. Women were less concerned with a man's appearance than with his social standing and ability to provide for a wife and children; but, to many women's frustration, in all of the thirty-seven cultures, men placed a high value on a woman's physical attractiveness and regarded attractiveness as much more important in choosing a mate than women did. This wasn't a difference that popped up only in the media-soaked United States but in all of the many different kinds of cultures sampled, all over the world. Something so consistent must be linked to human biology, not to the shifting sands of variable cultural beliefs. But *why* are men so focused on a woman's appearance?

Dev began with the basics. He knew that having more offspring is what drives evolution. That means that choosing your mate is the most important biological decision you make, since your chances of getting your genes into the next generation depend very strongly on the quality of your mate. A woman's health is certainly one element of that. But the evolutionary bottom line is her fertility: her ability to produce children. This means that in addition to reflecting her health, a woman's physical appearance should be very strongly connected with her ability to have many healthy children. So he looked for a link between woman's shape—her waist-hip ratio—and her ability to have children.

One link between her shape and fertility is estrogen. The female hormone, estrogen, lowers a woman's waist-hip ratio by causing more fat to be stored in her hips and thighs, and less in her waist. Because of these effects, a typical young woman in her late teens will have a waist-hip ratio of 72 percent: a waist size less than three-quarters as big as her hip size. A typical young man's ratio is 85 percent. (The waist size used for these ratios is the *smallest* waist rather than the "trouser" waist, which is measured just above the hips.) When a woman's estrogen level falls, as it does after her menopause, her waist-hip ratio goes up. Because estrogen is essential for a woman to become pregnant and governs how her fat is deposited, a woman's waist-hip ratio could show that she has enough estrogen to be fertile.

So lower waist-hip ratios might signal both health and fertility, but does having a lower ratio actually make women more attractive to men? One clue is the appearance of women that men pay to look at in magazines like *Playboy* or who are chosen for beauty contests like the Miss America pageant. It turns out that these women have waist-hip ratios that are much lower than average young women. A typical Playmate has a waist just 67 percent—two-thirds—the size of her hips.

To get a better idea of just how strong men's preference for low waist-hip ratios might be, Dev decided to set up an experiment. He began by making three drawings of a woman viewed from the front who was five feet, five inches tall and whose weight was 90, 120, or 150 pounds, so that one was "underweight," one "normal weight," and one "overweight." Next he made four drawings of each of the three with four different waist sizes so that the ratio of waist to hip varied from 70 to 100 percent. Then he asked his male psychology students to give an attractiveness score to each of the twelve drawings. The majority of the young men judged the woman weighing 120 pounds with the lowest waist-hip ratio of 70 percent to be the most attractive. Those who chose the lighter figure still preferred the lowest waist-hip ratio. So nearly all the men chose the lowest waist-hip ratio as the most attractive, regardless of the weight group they preferred.

When Dev published the results of his experiment in 1993, it attracted a lot of attention and set off a frenzy of more than a hundred other studies. Research groups all over the world wanted to find out if a similar preference for small waists and big hips would also be found in other places and cultures. Those who believed that attractiveness depended on cultural values were eager to prove Dev wrong. Psychologists and anthropologists trekked through jungles and across deserts so they could show his drawings to isolated groups of men in the most out-of-the-way places. And, while these men sometimes varied in how heavy they liked women to be, virtually all of them chose the figures whose waists were much smaller than their hips as the most attractive.

But one group seemed to be an exception. Among the Hadza hunter-gatherers, a group of a thousand people living in a remote area of northwest Tanzania, many of the men preferred larger waists when shown Singh's drawings of women viewed from the front. However, when they were later shown drawings of women viewed from the side rather than the front, Hadza men, like men pretty much everywhere, preferred the women with low waist-hip ratios. While some preferences may be culturally variable, a preference for women with low waist-hip ratios seems to be pretty universal among men.

What Are the Benefits of Lower Waist-Hip Ratios?

So men's preference for small waists and big hips seems to be quite well demonstrated, but what benefit are men getting when they select a partner with a low waist-hip ratio? Most researchers seemed content to show *what* men liked but not *why* they liked it. Many simply waved the "health and fertility" banner to explain the preference.

This is where we come in. The more we thought about these claims, the less convinced we were. True, women with higher waist-hip ratios do tend to be less healthy, but these negative health effects don't begin to show up until women reach their fifties and sixties, well past the age when they are having babies. So preferring a woman with a small waist-hip ratio does not promise a healthier mate during her childbearing years.

But even if women with low waist-hip ratios aren't healthier moms, perhaps they are more fertile, as the connection with estrogen might suggest. That would be a very good reason for men's preference because fertility—the ability to produce children—is the gold standard in evolution. However, when we look at women who have had babies, they almost always have *bigger* waists than women who have not been pregnant, and they have just as much estrogen. If a man is looking for a woman who has proven that she can have children, he should prefer a woman with a bigger waist.

But perhaps a low waist-hip ratio in a young woman is a sign of her future fertility. Fortunately, we were able to find a study that could shed some light on this possibility. Young women with fertility problems—women who would have difficulty getting pregnant without medical help—usually have irregular menstrual cycles or unusual bleeding patterns. Some Dutch researchers had wondered whether measuring waist-hip ratios could help physicians identify young women with these kind of problems. So they measured the waist and hip in several hundred women in their late teens and asked each of them to carefully describe her menstrual cycle and periods. If a waist-hip ratio predicts a young woman's fertility, those with irregular menstrual patterns should have higher ratios. But they found there was *no difference* in the waist-hip ratios of those with normal cycles and those with irregular cycles. If there was no difference, how could young men be using the waist-hip ratio as a clue to a woman's potential fertility?

What bothered us even more was that no one had suggested any *reason why* having a small waist and rounded hips should be connected to a woman's ability to have children. Researchers seemed to be regarding the ratio as a kind of mysterious sign or signal that was supposed to accidentally point to better health or fertility. But they didn't explain why having a lower waist-hip ratio should be beneficial to a young woman. If a woman's estrogen hormone tells her to store more fat in her hips and legs and less in her waist, as Singh argued, *why* does it do this?

Why Do Women Carry Their Weight in the Hips and Legs?

Young women have a lower waist-hip ratio than men because the women have both a smaller waist and *bigger* hips. So let's start there. What makes a woman's hips bigger? Although the bones in a woman's pelvis are a bit wider apart than a man's, the main difference is that women have much more fat covering their hips, buttocks, and legs than a man does. A typical young woman has a layer of fat more than an inch thick over her hips, buttocks, and legs; a man has less than a third of an inch. Because of this fatty layer, a woman's hip circumference is typically four inches larger than that of a man with the same height, giving the average woman fourteen pounds more fat in her legs than the average man. This thick layer of fat in the lower part of a woman's body is the main reason women have much more body fat than men.

Because of women's ample lower-body fat, when you compare young women with almost any other animal, even thin women have a surprisingly large amount and percentage of body fat. When Susan graduated from high school weighing just 118 pounds, she already had *thirty-five* pounds of body fat. That means that nearly *one-third* of her total body weight was fat! Most wild animals, including our close relatives among the monkeys and apes, have only about *5 percent* of their body weight as fat—one twentieth. It is difficult to find other animals that even approach a slim woman's level of 30 percent. Two that do come close are bears settling down to hibernate and whales swimming in arctic waters. Bears need extra fat to survive the long winter without feeding, and whales need a thick layer of fat to insulate their bodies from the frigid water. But why do slender young women need so much?

Women's fat is not just very unusual compared to other animals; it is also quite different from the fat men have. In contrast to a woman like the youthful Susan with thirty-five pounds of fat, a young man with the same height and weight would have less than fifteen pounds of fat. Where women have more fat, men have more muscle. And, of course, women's fat is also arranged quite differently than men's. While young women have most of their fat in their hips, buttocks, and legs, men carry most of their fat in their bellies, much like other animals.

There is little doubt that men find women's lower-body fat attractive. Two anthropologists at Emory University studied men's preferences in fifty-eight different cultures and found that men almost always preferred women with large or fat legs and hips. In many groups where food is limited, young women in their teens are kept apart and live in separate huts, where they are fed extra food so that their legs and hips become as plump as possible before they are married.

Recently R. Matthew Montoya, a young psychologist starting out at the University of North Carolina, wondered what specific areas of a woman's body were most important to men when they judge attractiveness. So he gave a group of male psychology students a list of twenty-one areas and asked them to rate the importance of each one in his ideal woman. Not unexpectedly, the men gave women's "chests" the highest rating, but the next three highest-rated areas, ranking just slightly below chests, were the buttocks, legs, and hips, the main areas where women store fat. Not only do women have very large amounts of fat in their hips, buttocks, and legs, but men find this fat especially appealing.

So what is it about the fat in a woman's lower body that might be connected with motherhood? Could it be the calories? One pound of fat has about four thousand calories, and it costs about sixty thousand extra calories to have a baby, so lower-body fat could be valuable for the calories it contains. But if the role of women's fat is just to supply calories, why don't the females of other mammals store as much fat as women for pregnancy and nursing? And why does it matter *where* women's fat is stored? Why should some fat be regarded as attractive, and some not? Waist fat has just as many calories as leg fat, yet men do not admire waist fat. Is there something else that might be important about lower-body fat?

Will was looking at waist, hip, and thigh measurements for American women with different numbers of children, and he noticed an unexpected difference in the location of their fat. He found that the more children a woman has, the less of her fat is in the lower part of her body—the fat in her hips, buttocks, and legs that men admire. This happens even though she has plenty to eat and is usually gaining weight. She may add some fat to this lower part of her body, but compared with her total amount of fat, there is less and less in her hips and thighs. This loss of fat seems to be connected to motherhood, because it is connected to the number of children a woman has had. This change in the location of women's fat will probably come as no surprise to women who have been dismayed to find that the fat in their thighs and buttocks seems to be migrating to their bellies after having children or to those who have employed plastic surgeons to move it back.

Since we found that this loss of fat is connected with motherhood and knowing that a woman's body undergoes many changes during pregnancy and nursing, we looked to see if this is the time when a woman's lower-body fat decreases. Sure enough, late in pregnancy and during nursing is when some of the fat in a woman's hips and thighs is lost. We were also surprised to discover that during these crucial stages of late pregnancy and nursing, a woman eats *less* than she needs and instead uses up some of the fat in her lower body. Why does she eat less when her baby is growing the most? If a woman were just storing fat for its calories, why wouldn't she just keep eating more the way she does earlier in her pregnancy rather than using up calories in her fat that might be needed later if times get bad?

In American mothers, the *share* of her fat that is in her lower body decreases each time she gives birth. In places where food supplies are limited, the total *amount* of a mother's lower-body fat will go down each time she has a baby, and she will end up much thinner by the time her periods stop, rather than gaining weight like American mothers. (These are the groups where men may prefer Dev's "overweight" sketches.) It seems as though something besides the calories in a woman's lower-body fat is used up during pregnancy and nursing even when she has plenty to eat. What could it be? What does a woman's stored fat have besides calories?

Omega-3 Fats and the Needy Brain

To answer this, we need to go back to the key issue we discussed in part 1: the difference between omega-6 and omega-3 fats. Omega-3 fats not only have beneficial effects on our weight and health, they also play a very critical role in our brains. If an infant mouse has plenty of omega-6 fat in its diet but very little omega-3, it will end up with a thinner brain that has fewer and smaller nerve cells; and there will be many fewer connections among its nerve cells. As a result, this unfortunate mouse has a hard time learning anything. Its brain is poorly developed because it has much less DHA, the most complex of the omega-3 fats. DHA makes up a third of the fatty membrane that encloses each nerve cell in our brains. It helps our 100 billion nerve cells to grow, send messages to each other, and form the thousands of connections each nerve cell makes with others that enable us to think. If all of the membranes in our nerve cells were spread out, they would cover more than five football or soccer fields; and one-third of every membrane is DHA!

Now we begin to see why human mothers have a much greater need for fat than other animals. In general, brain sizes follow body sizes. For example, whales and elephants have bigger brains than we do, to go along with their much bigger bodies. But our big brains are an exception to the rule; in fact, they are *seven times* larger than they should be for an animal our size. This means that we need a lot of DHA to build and run our gigantic brains. Just feeding our big brains takes a quarter of all the calories we use at rest, but DHA is much harder to come by. As our brains grew larger over human evolution, it became a greater and greater challenge to get the very large amount of DHA we needed to build and maintain such enormous brains.

Even small differences in the amount of DHA in the diet of a mother and her newborn child can make a difference to the development of the child's brain. Although women's breast milk has quite a bit of DHA, until recently most infant formulas did not include DHA, though they did contain some omega-3 alpha-linolenic. A number of studies have shown that babies fed either breast milk or formula with added DHA do better on mental and vision tests than infants fed formula without DHA. Other studies have shown that children also do better on mental tests when a mother has more DHA in her diet. In our own research, we have found that American children—especially girls—with higher levels of omega-3 in their diets score better on mental tests, while those with more omega-6 fat in their diets tend to have lower test scores. So babies' brains need lots of omega-3 DHA to work properly. If they receive less, their brains simply don't work as well.

From Mother to Child

From the day she was conceived, Susan's daughter Jessica—like all human babies—needed lots of DHA for her growing brain and body. In addition to the very high levels needed for the brain, there are also significant amounts of DHA in the blood, organs, and muscles. And until Jessica stopped nursing, all of that DHA had to come from Susan. And since Susan cannot make omega-3 fat, the DHA Jessica needed had to come either from what Susan was getting in her own diet or from what she had stored in her body. During the last trimester, when Jessica's brain was growing rapidly, she needed at least two drops (100 milligrams) a day of DHA—more than the amount in Susan's food. Moreover, after Jessica was born, her brain and body grew even faster, so that she needed even more DHA from Susan's milk—three drops (150 milligrams) a day. But Susan also needed DHA to keep her own brain and body running, ideally at least five drops (250 milligrams) a day. This might not seem like very much—two or three drops for Jessica and five for Susan—but DHA is quite scarce in our diet. Like the average American women, Susan gets just 70 milligrams of DHA in her daily diet, less than two drops, and much less than half of what she and her baby jointly need. So how can Susan come by all of the extra DHA she needs for Jessica?

The answer to this question tells us why women need fat and why men like women with generous hips and shapely legs. All mothers get the critical DHA for their babies from their own body fat—the fat stored away in their hips, buttocks, and legs. Regardless of how much omega-3 there may be in a mother's current diet, most of the DHA she gives to her baby comes from her lower-body fat—fat that has much more DHA than the fat in her waist. Other essential fatty acids needed by her baby also come from her stored fat.

This is why Susan eats less late in her pregnancy, when Jessica's brain is growing rapidly. Susan's body knows that she needs to take in fewer calories in order to begin dissolving some of her lower-body fat so that the DHA stored there can pass over to Jessica. The placenta that connects Jessica to her mother also has a special ability to transport DHA from Susan to Jessica. It can push DHA "uphill," creating a higher level of DHA in Jessica's blood than in her mother's. Once Susan is nursing Jessica, even more of Susan's fat dissolves to supply DHA for her baby, and she is delighted to find that her fat is melting away— nursing is the one time in a woman's life when it's really easy to lose weight.

It's easy for Susan to shed pounds when she is nursing because her body wants to break down fat in her hips, buttocks, and thighs to deliver some of its hoarded DHA to her baby. Without realizing it, she eats less than she needs so that this will happen. One pound of a mother's lower-body fat typically has about thirty-six drops of DHA (1,800 milligrams), though this amount depends on what she has been eating over time. A typical nursing mother breaks down close to two pounds of her body fat each month, and this frees up enough DHA to supply most of her baby's needs. So a mother with thirty pounds or more of stored fat, like Susan in her early twenties, has enough DHA deposited in her fat bank to supply the needs of several children.

It took Susan quite a long time to collect all of this extra DHA from her diet. She did it by setting up a kind of layaway account. When she was born, she already had a little more fat than a newborn boy, and she slowly accumulated the additional DHA she would need for her own children by putting aside a tiny amount each day in her lower-body fat stores. As Susan was growing up and making these small deposits each day into her fat savings account, they slowly added up. By her first birthday, she already had more lower-body fat and less waist fat than a typical boy. As she grew, this difference steadily increased, eventually giving her the characteristic hourglass shape of a young woman with a small waist and a large store of DHA in her lower-body fat.

Because of their greater need for DHA, girls (and women) also have a greater ability to concentrate DHA in their blood and body fat than boys and are better at making DHA from other, simpler omega-3 fats. They may also have higher levels of DHA in their own brains.

Once a young woman finishes growing, her lower-body fat savings account is locked up until she becomes pregnant. Even if she loses weight, her lower-body fat and the omega-3 it contains are usually protected.

Once we had the idea that a woman's lower-body fat holds the precious DHA needed for future babies, we wondered whether having more of this fat might affect when a girl has her first menstrual period. Surprisingly, there had been some disagreement about what triggers this important life change. Some claimed that a girl needs to have a certain total amount of body fat before she can start her periods, but others had disputed that. Given our new idea about where special brain-building fats are stored, we wondered whether the *location* of her fat might be more important than the total amount. If lower-body fat is a DHA bank, then girls with more lower-body fat will have more DHA in the bank and so can afford to start their periods earlier. We found, much to our delight, that they do. Girls with more lower-body fat do mature earlier, while girls with more waist fat mature later! (There are few things in science as satisfying as making a prediction that is supported by the evidence.) This helps to explain why girls in countries with limited food supplies may not have their first period until age seventeen or eighteen.

This led us to another, more surprising idea. If the fat stored in a mother's hips and legs provides omega-3 for her children's brains, and brains work better with more omega-3, then it seemed to us that women with more of their fat stored there—women with a lower waist-hip ratio—ought to have smarter children. So we looked for a connection between a mother's waist-hip ratio and how well her children scored on four tests relating to mental ability. Any effect that a mother's fat might have was not so easy to determine, because there is a strong genetic component to test scores and a strong relationship with the parents' education and mental ability. But even when we took these factors into account, the children of the mothers with more lower-body fat and less waist fat still scored better on the tests. Further supporting this connection between a woman's body shape and her omega-3, a recent study has shown that women with more lower-body fat and less waist fat have more omega-3 in their blood.

So now we can understand why young women need to have such a large amount of fat in their hips, buttocks, and legs compared with other animals and with their mates. Other animals have small brains, and men just need to maintain the brain their mother gave them—not make new brains, as women do. Women's lower-body fat functions as a DHA bank that takes in small deposits as a girl grows and matures, but only allows withdrawals during her last months of pregnancy and while she is nursing, when her infant's brain is growing rapidly. Because it is harder for an adult woman to replace the DHA her children have withdrawn from this bank, each child that she has tends to draw down from the fat savings account in her lower-body, and the amount of DHA in her blood tends to decrease with each pregnancy. In fact, a woman's brain can even shrink during her pregnancy in order to help provide more DHA to her baby.

This also explains why men find the thick layer of fat that envelopes a woman's hips, buttocks, and legs so attractive—because they "know" unconsciously and without being aware of it that this fat is valuable and can help their children have better brains.

Why a Woman's Need for DHA Can Cause Her to Gain Excess Weight

This critical role of women's fat in storing DHA for her children also helps to explain why the changes in our diets in recent decades have been causing American women to gain excess weight. In chapter 2 we saw that because American women have very high omega-6 and low omega-3 in their diets, they have much lower levels of DHA in their milk than women in other countries. Since most of the DHA in a woman's milk comes from her fat, this shows that American women also have lower percentages of DHA in their fat. The percentage of DHA in a woman's fat depends on the amount of DHA in her blood, and that, in turn, depends on the balance of omega-3 and omega-6 in her diet. The extremely unbalanced diet of American women results in a low level of DHA in their blood and a correspondingly low percentage in their stored fat. A woman with more omega-3 from her diet, like women in Japan, will have much more DHA in her blood, and a much higher percentage of DHA in her fat.

The lower the percentage of DHA in a woman's fat, the more fat she needs to have the same overall amount of DHA. If a woman gets half as much DHA from her diet as another woman, she will have half as much DHA in each pound of her fat. In order to have the same *total* amount of DHA in her fat stores, she will need to have twice as much fat as the woman with a diet high in omega-3. Because American women have such low levels of omega-3 from their diets, their bodies may be pushing them to store additional fat to help them provide the DHA they need for their babies' brains. Women with more DHA from their diet, like those in Japan and Europe, have less need to store such large amounts of fat and, as a result, will tend to be thinner than American women. This is another reason why eating a diet very high in omega-6 and low in omega-3 may cause American women to gain excess weight.

We now have one big piece of the puzzle of why women need fat. Our brains are much bigger than those of other apes, but this advance isn't free. One major cost is an increased demand for the DHA needed to build our giant brain. Women, as mothers, need to have large amounts of these fats in reserve because their daily diets don't contain enough to supply their infants' rapidly growing brains. A woman's hips and thighs are her principal bank for these brain-essential fats. That's why men prefer women with bigger hips: Generous hips promise brainy children. But what message does the other part of a waist-hip ratio, the small waist, convey? That is the mystery we will explore next, as young women have to encounter yet another very high cost of having a big brain.

CHAPTER 4

The Mystery of the Tiny Waist

B rian, a nineteen-year-old student at York University in England, is seated a few feet away from a seventeen-inch color monitor, his eyes fixed on a small black cross at the center of the screen. Brian is not playing the latest video game; he is a volunteer in a psychology experiment. As he watches, a photograph of a young woman briefly flashes on the screen. Her face is blurred, but not her body. Standing facing the camera, arms at her sides and feet slightly apart, she is wearing a semitransparent, flesh-colored bra and panties. After her image disappears, Brian has to indicate how attractive he finds her by entering a number from one to nine on a keypad; he taps the five key. But this is only a small part of what this experiment is really about.

During the two seconds that the woman's image is on the screen, a sensitive digital camera mounted below the monitor photographs Brian's eyes one hundred times. Just as our eyes always do, Brian's eyes rapidly dart around so that he can aim the sharpest part of his retina at the areas that interest him the most. Without any conscious effort on his part, his brain knits this jumble of separate sharp images together into a seamless image of the woman. Meanwhile, the digital record of his rapid eye movements reveals exactly where he is looking while he is evaluating female beauty.

You might guess that Brian would look first at the woman's breasts, but that's not what happens. Like almost all of the male subjects in this experiment, Brian looks first at her *waist*. As his eyes zoom around the photograph, he does get around to looking at her chest, but he spends almost as much time looking at her waist. And there is nothing special about this particular photograph or about Brian. His eye movements are typical of the way that he and the other volunteers look at the photographs of forty-two female undergraduates. The eye-tracking equipment says that waists rule.

The experiment that Brian volunteered for is yet another salvo in a long and hard-fought scientific battle about what aspect of a woman's body is most important to men's judgments of her attractiveness. On one side is Dev Singh and his view that a woman's waist-hip ratio is most important. On the other side is a research group headed by Martin Tovee, a psychologist at Newcastle University in northern England, and his idea that it is a woman's BMI that is most important, her weight in relation to her height. (Women's faces and personalities are even more important in men's judgments of attractiveness, but they are not part of this debate.)

The eye-tracking experiment is an ingenious new method that Tovee devised to advance his BMI argument. But, as in Tovee's other studies of attractiveness, this experiment does have one peculiar aspect. None of the men rate any of the forty-two young women in the photographs as very attractive. While they do rate the women with BMIs below 20 as more attractive than the heavier women, none are rated very high. Brian's highest rating is only five out of a possible nine, and Brian is no pickier than the other volunteers. So what is it that Brian is looking for as his eyes dart around the young woman's waist? Why is her waist the first thing that he looks at? And why are none of the women in the photographs very appealing to him?

To help answer these questions, we can ask what it would take to make Brian punch the nine key. Lindsey Vuolo, Kimberly Phillips, Jamie Edmundson, and Kira Milan are also university students, like the young women in Tovee's photographs, but they are not so typical. All four were recently selected as *Playboy* magazine Playmates of the Month. For posterity, each Playmate reports her height, weight, waist, hip, and bust measurements. To see how they differ from average students, we can compare the measurements of more than six hundred Playmates with those taken from three hundred undergraduate women at a California university. So how does an average student differ from a typical Playmate?

Many people guess that the Playmates have larger bust sizes than typical undergraduates but, surprisingly, they don't. The students actually have larger bust sizes (on average, one inch larger). So where else should we look? One big difference is that Playmates tend to be slimmer. Their average BMI is just 18 compared to 22 for the typical California undergraduate, supporting Tovee's argument that lower BMIs are more attractive. For women with the same height, this amounts to a weight difference of about twenty pounds.

But what if we only compare the Playmates with those California undergrads whose BMIs match theirs? This leaves us with a quarter of the students. Now we find that the low-BMI students and Playmates have nearly identical hip sizes, but the Playmates' waist sizes still average *four inches* smaller than the students'! This is a huge difference. The Playmates have about the same amount of fat in their hips, buttocks, and legs as the slimmer students do, but much less fat in their waists. So having a really small waist seems to be what sets women rated as very attractive apart from more typical young women who have equally low BMIs.

Men seem to like small waists, but just how small would they like them to be? A real woman's waist size cannot dip too low, because there has to be room for her internal organs. But what if there were no limits? There is actually a way to answer this curious question. Artists who draw women characters for comics, animated films, graphic novels, or computer games do not have to give them ribs, intestines, livers, and spleens, so they can make the women they draw look any way they want as long as they are attractive to the men who buy their products.

We decided to find out which of these imaginary women are the most attractive to men and to see what those women are like. We recruited some university students in California to help, and almost five hundred responded to our request for "an image of the most attractive imaginary woman" they could think of. For each image, we measured the width of the waist and hip, and then divided the waist by the hip size to determine the ratio.

For typical flesh-and-blood California coeds, the waist size is almost three-quarters of the hip size. Playmates' much smaller waists are only two-thirds as big as their hips. But for the imaginary women, while the hip size is normal, the average waist is just *half* the size of the hips! It gets better. The single most popular imaginary woman, chosen by more students than any other, was Jessica Rabbit from the film *Who Framed Roger Rabbit?* Her waist size is a mere *one-third* the size of her hips. And there is independent evidence of her popularity: She was also chosen the "Sexiest Cartoon Character of All Time" in a contest sponsored by Cadbury's. So, when men are no longer limited by what is anatomically possible, they seem to prefer waists that are half the size of *Playboy* models'. So why do they have such a strong preference for young women with tiny waists?

A number of researchers thought it might be helpful if we knew what is going on inside men's brains when they look at nude photographs of small-waisted women considered to be attractive. They felt that this was an important scientific question to answer using multimillion-dollar, state-of-the-art brain-scanning equipment. They found that looking at nude pictures of women with low waist-hip ratios lights up the same pleasure centers in men's brains that are activated by cocaine, heroin, or other addictive drugs. And based on Tovee's eye-tracking experiment, we know that these men are spending a lot of their time looking at the models' waists. So it seems that evolution has programmed men to respond strongly and positively to small-waisted women. But this still doesn't tell us why.

If you ask Brian why he spends so much time looking at the women's waists in the photographs or why he finds very small waists attractive, he doesn't have a clue. Men just don't know why they like this female shape. That is because the answer lies in the "adaptive uncon-scious," the subject of Malcolm Gladwell's popular book *Blink*. The adaptive unconscious is the large part of our minds that operates with-out our knowing what it is doing—or why—and that has been shaped by evolution to keep us alive and to help us have as many healthy chil-dren as possible. Just as we do not stop to think about what to do when we see a car bearing down on us, we do not think about why we have a preference for a certain body shape.

But there is always a reason that makes evolutionary sense. Why does a full belly feel good? Because you need to eat to live. Why is sex enjoyable? So that we have children. Why is parenting rewarding? To help our children and our genes survive. So, why should men have a built-in attraction to small-waisted women? It must be very strongly connected to a woman's success in having children. Women with small waists must have a better chance of having healthy babies; otherwise men's small-waist preference would make no sense.

An Extremely Troubling Puzzle

So what does a young woman's waist size tell us? First, her waist size is very strongly related to her BMI. You cannot have a small waist size without also having a low BMI. Playmates have low BMIs, and when we compare students with Playmates, the few students with BMIs less than 18 come close to having the same tiny waist size as the Playmates. When Brian is asked to judge how much body fat the women in the photographs have, he looks only at the waist.

And most young women, at least until recently, also have pretty low BMIs. In the early 1970s, eight thousand American women of all ages were asked, "What's the least you've weighed since you turned eighteen?" Almost all had their lowest weight between the ages of eighteen and twenty, and the average of these low weights was 117 pounds. Almost two-thirds had a BMI of 17 to 19, on the low side of the range that Tovee's studies have found men most prefer. And though most young women do not have waist sizes as small as Playmates, the young women with the lowest BMIs are the ones that naturally come the closest. Since men's preferences and young women's bodies are similar, having a low BMI and small waist must be very beneficial.

So what do we know about the connection between a woman's BMI and her ability to have babies? It's exactly the opposite of what it should be! Women with BMIs well below 20—like Playmates, the women men prefer in Tovee's studies, and the students with the smallest waists—tend to be *less* healthy, *less* fertile, and *less* able to conceive children. Women athletes or ballet dancers with BMIs this low often stop having periods and are unable to have children until they gain some weight.

This is very disconcerting. We know that men prefer the appearance of women with extremely small waists and that looking at mere photos of thin-waisted women sparks their pleasure centers. But if such women are less fertile and less healthy than heavier women, how can we explain such a powerful preference in men? This question was keeping us up at night, because it made no evolutionary sense. Above all else, evolution operates relentlessly to select only those that are the best at reproducing. Yet thinner women seem to be worse at reproducing than heavier women. Why should men be endowed with a preference for women who are *less* good at reproducing? How could that kind of preference ever evolve? The answer, it turns out, lies in something that happens to an American woman every two minutes—though, fortunately for them, its consequences are well concealed by modern medicine.

Hidden in Plain Sight

Marcie is tired and discouraged as she begins her twenty-second hour of labor: Why is her son taking so long to be born? Marcie is twenty-eight years old, of average height (five feet, four inches), and, at 150 pounds with a BMI of 26, was slightly "overweight" when she began her first pregnancy. Marcie is determined to experience a "natural childbirth." She remembers quite well the many times in her prenatal classes she held an ice cube in her hand for sixty seconds while taking deep breaths. But her contractions have been much more painful and have gone on for much longer than she ever imagined. Now, as she waits for the results of her ultrasound, she is wondering how much longer this can go on.

The ultrasound is not encouraging. Her doctor tells her that her son is not moving down her birth canal. She explains that like many first-time mothers, Marcie has "obstructed labor" because her son's head is too big to pass through her birth canal, and this means Marcie needs to have a Cesarean section (or C-section) to deliver her baby. She tells Marcie that her problem is not unusual and that one in three first-time mothers have their babies delivered in this way. After an anesthetic is injected into Marcie's spine, her doctor quickly makes an opening in the tense skin of her belly, and then in the wall of her womb. She reaches in and lifts out Marcie's eight-pound baby boy, Michael, crying vigorously as he takes his first breaths of air. The pediatrician looks him over and pronounces him completely healthy and normal.

Just as Marcie's doctor has told her, her situation is not at all unusual: These same events unfold some seven hundred times a day in American hospitals, as first-time mothers like Marcie have their babies by C-section. We can almost hear the voice of an officious policeman saying, "Move along, people, there is nothing to see here." And yet, if we think about it, what we are saying is that one of three first-time American mothers is unable to deliver her baby through her birth canal and needs to have it brought out instead through a surgical incision. Whatever happened to Mother Nature? What's wrong with the "birth canal"? And what happens to first-time mothers when C-sections are not available?

When C-sections Are Not an Option

Six thousand miles away, on her bed in her home in a small village in the African country of Niger, Fatimata Ataher, a much smaller young woman than Marcie, is in the third day of her first labor. But unlike Marcie, Fatimata has no doctor to help her. Like most women in her country, she is giving birth without medical assistance. When her son is finally born late on the third day of her labor, he does not cry or take a breath. Like Marcie's son, Fatimata's son was too big to fit through her birth canal, but, unfortunately, having a surgical delivery was not an option for her.

Fatimata is lucky to survive her pregnancy; in Niger, one woman in seven dies in childbirth compared with one in five thousand American mothers, and several other countries have similarly high rates of deaths in mothers. Obstructed labor and the bleeding or infection that often accompany it account for most of these deaths. And even when mothers like Fatimata do survive their many days of labor, very few of their babies are born alive. (Many of the babies that are born alive also die within a few days because of birth-related injuries.) Clearly, obstructed labor is a major cause of difficulty and death for both mothers and infants.

But Fatimata's suffering does not end with the loss of her son. Because of the pressure of his head on the tissues above and below her birth canal during the three days of her labor, she develops a fistula, a devastating and incapacitating problem that affects about two hundred thousand mothers in her country and as many as three and a half million women worldwide. Fatimata decides to make the long journey from her village to the capital city of Niamey, where the National Hospital is located, and joins the "women of the courtyard" who live on the hospital grounds while waiting for surgical teams from abroad to arrive. When Njoki Nganga, an obstetrical nurse volunteer from New Jersey, first saw the women gathered there, it was a life-changing experience for her: "No words can adequately describe the waves of emotion that overcame me when I met the women of the courtyard for the first time." Njoki is now the nursing director for the International Organization for Women and Development, the group that sponsored her trip to Niger and which also sponsored the surgical team that successfully repaired Fatimata's fistula and gave her back her life.

But while the terrible consequences of obstructed labor today are found mainly in Africa and South Asia, not so long ago they confronted first-time mothers everywhere, and young women looked forward to their first pregnancy with a mixture of anticipation and dread.

Investigating Childbirth in Nineteenth-Century Sweden

Thirty years ago, Dr. Ulf Högberg was a young Swedish physician providing medical care in rural Mozambique. While serving there, he saw several young mothers die in childbirth. Even today, he describes this as "the most ugly part of clinical work I have been part of," and the experience had a profound effect on him. The Sweden he had grown up in had a well-organized, state-run health care system and was known as one of the healthiest countries in the world. The infant death rate was very low and very few mothers died in childbirth. But after his experiences in Africa, Dr. Högberg wondered what things had been like for Swedish mothers before modern obstetrics was available, and he teamed up with a colleague, Goran Brostrom, to try to find out.

They realized that because Swedish clergymen in the 1800s had kept very detailed records for their parishes, they might find the answer there. They looked at the birth and death records for women in seven typical parishes over a one-hundred-year period. Although they were expecting that childbirth might be a factor in women's deaths, they were still surprised to find that one married woman in fourteen died in childbirth! In fact, childbirth accounted for half of the deaths of women under fifty, most due to obstructed labor and related bleeding and infections following delivery. This shows us what the dangers of obstructed labor were like just a few hundred years ago. But an anthropologist with a love of bones, Larry Angel, has given us an even broader picture of the life-and-death consequences of childbirth during the long history of our species.

Investigating Childbirth in Europe, 30,000 BC to AD 1900

In 1980, two Delaware police detectives drove to the Smithsonian Institution in Washington with a skeleton in the trunk of their car. They wanted to show it to Larry Angel, the anthropologist known in CSI circles as "Sherlock Bones." Although his real job was curator of physical anthropology, in charge of the twenty-nine thousand human skeletons in the Smithsonian Institution's collection, Larry was the guy the FBI consulted when they needed the help of someone who could read skeletons the way the rest of us read a newspaper. After carefully examining the bones, Angel told the detectives that they had belonged to a very athletic young woman in her late teens or early twenties who played a wind instrument and who had been murdered at least eight months earlier. Angel's information enabled the detectives to identify the victim as twenty-year-old Susan Spahn, a college athlete and clarinet player, who had been missing for the past fourteen months. She was one of more than four hundred murder victims Angel helped the FBI to identify.

Larry Angel was the son of an English sculptor and as a child had been fascinated by the human skeleton his father kept in his studio. In college at Harvard, he started out studying classics but soon switched over to anthropology "because books just couldn't explain why human beings were the way they were." To find out why, he learned to read the bones they had left behind. His approach was monumental in scope: He examined and measured almost three thousand human skeletons of men and women from Europe dating from thirty thousand years ago through the nineteenth century and discovered a remarkably consistent pattern. First, he found that from the Stone Age to the nineteenth century, a typical woman died in her thirties, with many dying at younger ages. But, quite surprisingly, he also found that men typically died five years later than women. Five years may not seem like much, but this is exactly how long American women now outlive American men. What makes Angel's finding even more remarkable is that men are much more likely to die early from violence, injuries, infections, and blood vessel diseases than women. The only possible explanation he could come up with for men outliving women over these many centuries is that a great many women were dying in childbirth. So this is additional strong evidence that bearing children has been a very serious challenge for women during the two-hundred-thousand-year history of our species. It also tells us that the recent widespread use of C-sections for women with labor problems has been very important in helping women to live longer.

The Oldest Written Story

Although not quite as ancient a testimony to the perils of childbirth as some of the bones examined by Larry Angel, the first story ever written down also tells of the difficulty many women have delivering their babies. This is the ancient Mesopotamian story of Atrahasis, written more than five thousand years ago. The story relates how the gods created the first men and women to dig the canals needed for growing crops, but they were soon sorry because these pesky creatures were too fruitful, had too many children, and made too much noise, which was keeping the gods awake at night. To deal with this infestation, the gods sent a series of famines and plagues to reduce the human population to a more manageable size. In the fifth of these plagues, the goddess of childbirth turned away from mankind and "the womb was too tight to let a baby out." Finally, the gods sent a great flood to destroy mankind; but one man, Atrahasis, was told by a renegade god to make a boat, like Noah, and he and his family survived the flood. But to help limit the number of people in the future, the "womb-goddess Nintu" decreed that one-third of women would henceforth have difficulty giving birth: "the woman who gives birth, yet does not give birth success-fully." This is one more example of an abundance of evidence from the past that a great many women have had desperate problems giving birth through a birth canal that is often "too tight to let the baby out."

Why Are So Many of Our Babies Too Big?

The answer to this life-threatening puzzle is really quite simple: Many babies' heads are simply too big to pass through their mother's birth canal. And most babies who do make it through are just barely able to fit through the space enclosed by their mother's pelvic bones, a pas-sageway that is often smaller than the baby's head. But how did this come to be?

In 2002 the staff at the Kansas City Zoo set up a video camera in the cage of a pregnant orangutan they called Jill to film her labor and birth. In the video we see Jill, an auburn-haired, human-size ape sleep-ing peacefully on her side. She stirs, wakes up, lies there for a bit, then stands up, reaches down, and gently pulls out and lifts up her brand-new daughter, later named Josie. Josie is soon climbing onto her mother and holding tightly to her fur. What could be easier than having your first baby? Compare Jill's tranquil five-minute birth with Fatimata's three days of unsuccessful labor.

There are two reasons why giving birth is so much harder and so much more dangerous for us than for our ape cousins like Jill: Our brains are three times larger than theirs *and* we have pelvic bones that have been reshaped so that we can walk on our hind legs. The change in the pelvis came first, beginning about 6 million years ago when some pioneering apes first started walking upright. Walking this way required the pelvic bones to twist into a different shape, which also happened to make the birth canal smaller. That didn't bother the first upright-walking apes because they still had small brains. Even if their pelvis was now less roomy, their small-brained, small-headed babies could still pass through easily. But when the brains of our ancestors started to get bigger several million years later, a pelvis built for walking upright made it increasingly difficult for their brainier infants to fit through the birth canal. Our story would have been over right then if we had not evolved a number of ways to help our babies' big brains fit through pelvic bones streamlined for walking upright.

If we compare Susan's daughter Jessica just after she was born with the orangutan newborn Josie, one difference is that Jessica's skull bones are not joined together and can overlap each other during birth while Josie's skull bones are cemented together into a solid dome of bone. Having a collapsible skull helps Jessica squeeze through the parts of Susan's birth canal that are smaller than her head.

There is another even bigger change in what is inside Jessica's skull when she is born. Although she will end up with a much bigger brain than Josie, Jessica's brain has done much less of its growing when she is born. Some of the DHA that would have been used for her brain if it had grown more is stored instead in her slippery, squeezable fat. This explains why our newborn babies are much fatter than those of any other animal, even newborn harbor seals that have to swim in icy water soon after they are born.

Being born with a less-developed brain makes Jessica's birth easier, but it also means that she is quite helpless when she is born. While Josie can hold on to her mother's fur and support her own weight within a few hours of her birth, the best Jessica can do is to grasp her mother's finger for a few moments. It will take Jessica at least a year to catch up to Josie's newborn abilities. But despite the changes in our infants' skulls and the slowing down of their brain growth, there was still not enough room in the birth canal. Mothers had to change, too.

One thing that mothers had to do was to get taller, because a taller woman has a larger pelvis and more room for her babies to pass through. While ape mothers like Jill are typically half the size of their mates, women are much closer in height to theirs. Even today, short women, like Fatimata in Niger, are much more likely to have obstructed labor than taller women.

Another thing that helps us with our births is that a mother's strong contractions over many hours can loosen the ligaments joining her pelvic bones together and actually pry them apart to make her birth canal a little larger. Larry Angel could tell how many children a woman had had simply by looking at the changes and scars in her pelvic bones. But besides getting taller and having a somewhat expandable pelvis, the other way a young woman can keep her first child from growing too large before birth is to be thin and have a small waist. Let's see how that works.

Goldilocks and the Three Births

We have seen that Marcie had to have a surgical delivery in order for her son Michael to be born. When she conceived Michael, Marcie weighed 150 pounds. This is about twenty-five pounds more than typical first-time mothers a generation ago, and heavier than three-fourths of new mothers. Michael weighed eight pounds when he was born, heavier than three out of four first babies. Could there be a connection between Marcie's and Michael's heavier weight?

As sometimes happens, Marcie and her friend Ellen became pregnant at almost the same time. But Ellen weighed only ninety-five pounds when she conceived her daughter Melissa. Unlike Marcie's labor, Ellen's was very quick and easy for a first birth, lasting less than four hours. For her, natural childbirth was the perfect choice. But the reason that her labor was so easy was that her baby was quite small, weighing only four pounds. Because Melissa was so small, she had to spend her first two weeks in the special-care nursery.

When Susan conceived her daughter Jessica, she weighed 120 pounds, lighter than Marcie but heavier than Ellen, and fairly typical of first-time mothers at the time. And while her sixteen hours of labor seemed like a very long time to her, it is actually quite average for a first labor. Jessica was a typical seven-pound newborn girl and was born without any special assistance.

For Marcie, Ellen, and Susan, there seems to be a strong link between the mother's weight and her child's weight: the heavier the mother, the bigger the baby. And this same kind of connection is generally found between mothers and their newborn infants. How much a mother weighs when she becomes pregnant is strongly linked to how big her baby will be. This strong link between a mother's weight before pregnancy and her baby's birth weight has been found in more than a hundred different research studies.

But what about how much a woman eats *during* her pregnancy? Marcie and Ellen often went out to eat together after their prenatal classes. Marcie was surprised to find that her petite friend was eating more than she was, just the opposite of what usually happened before they became pregnant. And this is not at all unusual. Heavier mothers like Marcie tend to eat *less* during pregnancy but still have much bigger babies than the thinner mothers like Ellen, who eat more while they are pregnant. Though you might think that the mothers who gain the most weight during pregnancy would have the biggest babies, how much a mother eats *before* she becomes pregnant is more important than how much she eats during her pregnancy. The heavier she is before, the bigger her baby is likely to be. Mothers like Marcie who have eight-pound babies usually weigh thirty to forty pounds more when they become pregnant than mothers whose babies weigh only five or six pounds.

Because of this strong link between a mother's and baby's weight, a heavier first-time mother like Marcie is much more likely to have a baby that is too big for her birth canal. A very thin mother like Ellen has less than one chance in a hundred of an obstructed labor and only a small chance of needing a C-section. But a heavier mother like Marcie is ten times more likely to have obstructed labor and seven times more likely to need a C-section, and half of first-time mothers who are obese need a surgical delivery. But if a bigger baby like Marcie's son Michael is able to be born, he will usually be much stronger, hardier, and healthier than a small baby like Ellen's daughter Melissa.

So during most of human history it has been best for a first-time mother if she is not too heavy or not very thin. Susan is the just-right mom. Her baby is small enough to have a good chance of getting born but big enough to have a good chance of surviving after birth.

The Waist Is the Key

We've seen that a mother's weight and BMI help determine how big her baby is. But what does that have to do with men like Brian focusing on women's waists? The answer is this: A woman's waist fat is what mainly determines whether her baby will be too big. Women with bigger waists in relation to their hips are at greater risk. Typical young women have low weights and very little waist fat. But when a young woman weighs more than 140 pounds, more of her added fat goes to her waist, which is why a woman like Marcie is more likely to have a baby that is too big. The more waist fat she has, the greater her risk. Having a lower weight *and* less waist fat helps a woman to have a baby that is small enough to be born.

So one reason that young women tend to be thin and to have small waists before their first pregnancy is that small-waisted first-time mothers—and their babies—are more likely to survive labor. This unconscious understanding is built into men's brains, even though they don't know it's there. Those men in the past who linked up with smaller-waisted young women were more likely to have wives and children who survived. And those children have passed their father's preferences for smaller waists down to us.

"A woman cannot be too rich or too thin," Wallis Simpson famously said, but when it comes to men's judgments of women's attractiveness, this is not correct. When women are asked to predict how men will rate the attractiveness of women with different figures, most women think that the men will prefer thinner women than they actually do. It is a small waist combined with quite a bit of fat in the hips, buttocks, and thighs that men respond to. For, as we have seen, lower-body fat holds the key to bigger brains. That is why most men find super-skinny fashion models like Kate Moss much less attractive than Playmates. And because Playmates are also taller and have longer legs than average, despite having a low BMI and very low waist size, the average Playmate will still have thirty-two pounds of fat, just a bit less than Susan did in her early twenties.

Putting this all together, we were finally able to answer the question that was troubling us: why young women tend to be thinner than older women with children. Women need to keep their first babies small enough to be born. Being fairly thin and small-waisted along with broad hips is the best way to do that. Men prefer women that are more likely to have more surviving children. So Mother Nature has given young women a built-in tendency to have small waists combined with ample lower-body fat, and young men a built-in desire for this hourglass shape in their partners. But this is not quite the whole story. Now we need to look at what happens to women's waists after they have their first baby, why they change, and what this signals. This will help us to uncover two more reasons why men prefer women with smaller waists and another reason why it is better for first-time mothers to be thin.

CHAPTER 5

Why Waistlines Expand

Of all of the sixty-eight pounds of fat in Susan's body, those that she likes the least are spread around her waist and inside her belly. It seems to her that when she gains weight, most of it settles in her waist, which is just where she doesn't want it. In a dark corner of her basement are some rusting metal contraptions that were supposed to make her waist get smaller, and there are several books gathering dust on a shelf that claimed to have the secret for shrinking waists by many inches in just a few weeks. But neither the devices nor the books have made any difference. As she has gained weight, her waist has grown even faster.

A good part of the $40 billion American women spend each year trying to lose weight is aimed at their waists. Hardly a week goes by without a flood of advertising trumpeting some new foolproof device, diet, or method that guarantees a slimmer waist and "tighter abs." Many women go even further to attain a smaller waist. In 2008, for example, 310,000 American women had fat surgically removed from their waist area with liposuction, while another 143,000 had surgical "tummy tucks." It's easy to understand why. We've seen how men focus their attention on waists, and what tiny waists models and celebrities flaunt. So why do women add more to their waists than to other parts of their body as they gain weight?

Having a first baby seems to trigger a big change in how much women weigh and where a woman's fat goes when she gains weight. When Susan became pregnant with her son David, four years after Jessica was born, she had eight more pounds of fat than when she conceived Jessica. A big part of this new fat went to her waist, enlarging it by four inches. When a young woman weighs more than 140 pounds, like Marcie, more of the added weight goes to her waist than her hips. But for a woman who has already had a child, an even larger share of any weight she gains is added to her waist.

As we saw in the last chapter, the more waist fat a mother has when she starts her pregnancy, the bigger her baby is likely to be at birth. Susan's twenty-six-inch waist when she became pregnant with Jessica meant that she had enough waist fat to support the growth of a seven-pound baby. Because of Susan's height and pelvic size, a baby Jessica's size could squeeze through her birth canal. But when Susan became pregnant with David, her increased fat allowed David to be a pound heavier than Jessica when he was born, much more than the usual three-ounce difference between newborn boys and girls.

But wasn't this risky for Susan and David? Didn't his larger size make him more likely to get stuck during birth, like Marcie's eight-pound son, Michael? No, it didn't. Even though David was the same size as Michael, Susan's labor with him was four hours shorter than with Jessica. Thanks to Jessica's trailblazing, Susan's risk of obstructed labor was actually much smaller for her second birth even though her baby was much bigger. Giving birth to a first baby expands a woman's birth canal, so she can afford to have a bigger second child. As we saw earlier, Larry Angel could tell how many times a woman had given birth by seeing how much her pelvic bones had been pushed apart. Each of a woman's babies expands her birth canal, so that her next baby can safely be bigger.

Having a bigger baby is very desirable because bigger babies do much better than smaller ones. They are stronger, healthier, heavier, taller, and less prone to infections; they grow faster after birth; and they are more likely to survive infancy and childhood. Even with modern hospital care, a seven-pound baby like Jessica is almost one and a half times more likely to die in her first year of life than an eight-pound baby like her brother, David. American babies weighing eight to ten pounds have the smallest chances of dying. Even with special infant care, a six-pound newborn is almost three times more likely to die in infancy than one in the optimal eight-to-ten-pound range.

So if a mother adds weight and expands her waist after she has a baby, this extra weight is very likely to benefit her next child. The increased health and survival of bigger babies is why a woman with a child typically gains more weight in her twenties, gains a little less in her thirties, and her weight gain then tapers off. She gains the most weight during her childbearing years, when it can be most beneficial to her children. But she can only gain weight and have bigger, healthier children if she has enough food available to make this possible. In America we tend to take having plenty of food for granted. But when food is limited, as it still is in many countries, mothers cannot afford to have bigger children.

Yasmin, Jemelah, and Amir

Yasmin is a twenty-six-year-old mother of two living in rural Bangladesh, and she has much less to eat than Susan. Because her country suffers frequent flooding and droughts and has a very large number of people to feed for its size, food tends to be in short supply. Yasmin has a bit more than half as many calories in her daily diet as Susan. Typical of mothers in her country, Yasmin is six inches shorter than an average American woman, weighs ninety pounds, and has about sixteen pounds of body fat, less than half as much fat as Susan had at age eighteen.

Unlike Susan, Yasmin is likely to lose both weight and fat with each of her pregnancies and to become thinner each time she has a child. Her first child, her daughter Jemelah, weighed five pounds at birth. And her son Amir, despite being a boy, weighed the same as his sister. Half of all newborns in Bangladesh weigh less than five and a half pounds compared with one in twelve American babies. Being so small makes them much more vulnerable. Compared with American babies, children in Bangladesh are nine times more likely to die in their first five years, and they are especially vulnerable to infections.

But being small is not *all* bad. Because Amir and Jemelah are much smaller than a typical American baby, they require less nourishment from their mother before they are born and while they are nursing. And this is fortunate because she has much less that she can afford to give them. Amir and Jemelah will grow up to be smaller adults, like their mother, and this will help them to be better suited for life in a place where there is less food. If they were bigger, they would have had great difficulty passing through their mother's smaller birth canal and would be more likely to die of malnutrition, since bigger bodies require more calories to live and grow.

The genetic program passed down to us from our ancestral grandmothers helps mothers and children to be as big as their local food supply allows: bigger where food is abundant, as in the United States, and smaller in places like Bangladesh. As food supplies improve, bigger infants are born and grow into bigger adults. Four hundred years ago, Susan's ancestral grandmothers were the same size as Yasmin. Our genes prepare us to make the best of our local food supply by helping us to grow as big as we can for the amount of food that we have.

How Bigger Waists Make Bigger Babies

Dev Singh's doctor believed that having a larger waist and waist-hip ratio is less healthy for a woman because it increases the amount of sugar and fat (triglycerides) in her blood, her blood pressure, and her white blood cell activity. High blood sugar can lead to diabetes. Higher levels of triglycerides, blood pressure, and white cell activity all contribute to an increased risk of heart disease and stroke in some people. But these are also *exactly* the things that help mothers have bigger babies and survive childbirth. So how do they make babies bigger? It's all in the brain.

More than seventy years ago, two researchers at Northwestern University found that making a tiny cut deep inside the brain of a rat caused it to eat ravenously and become very fat. The rats who had this procedure were so desperate to eat when they awoke after the surgery, they literally inhaled their food. The part of the brain the researchers had cut into was the hypothalamus, an ancient part of the brain that controls most of the basic functions of our bodies, including eating.

Ten years later, researchers at the Jackson Laboratory in Bar Harbor, Maine, happened to notice an extremely fat mouse waddling around among its much thinner littermates and decided to find out what made it so fat. At first, they thought that there might be something wrong with its hypothalamus, but that was working just fine. After further investigation, they found that these mice had two bad copies of a certain gene, which they called the "obese" gene; but it took more than thirty years to find out just what that gene did. It turned out to be the gene that tells fat cells how to make a hormone called leptin. The more fat you have, the more leptin your fat cells make. Because a fat mouse could not make any leptin, its hypothalamus was convinced that it had no fat at all, so it kept telling it to eat as much as possible in order to get some fat. Also, despite being very fat, the female mice with no leptin were unable to have any offspring. Believing that they had no fat, their hypothalamus had turned off their reproductive systems. But if researchers gave them some leptin, their fertility was instantly restored.

Like those of other animals, Susan's fat cells also make leptin, and her leptin level strongly reflects the total amount of fat stored in her body. The more fat she has stored, the more leptin her hypothalamus finds in her blood. Her hypothalamus is an almond-size lump of nerve cells buried deep inside her brain; it is like the building supervisor for her body. One of its many jobs is to oversee Susan's reproductive functions, to make sure that she has the resources she needs to become pregnant and nurse her children so her children are the right size. It is especially interested in how much leptin is in Susan's blood because this shows the size of the fat stores, and it wants to be sure she has enough.

When she was growing up, her hypothalamus wanted Susan to have quite a bit of fat before it would allow her to start her menstrual cycle. When she was twelve and her fat level reached twenty-eight pounds, enough so that her leptin was six units, her hypothalamus decided that she had enough fat to start having periods. If her leptin level had not reached this level, as happens with some girls who train as gymnasts, her periods would have been delayed. Because Yasmin had much less fat when she was in her teens, her hypothalamus did not allow her to start having menstrual periods until she was seventeen. If Susan's fat level had later dropped to twenty-four pounds and her leptin level to five units, as it did for her athletic friend Natalie, her hypothalamus would have stopped her menstrual cycle until she regained the lost fat.

Her hypothalamus wants to know just how much fat she has stored, because her fat has the omega fats that her brain, body, and children will need. And the amount of fat she has also tells her hypothalamus about her food supply. The more fat she has, the more food she must have to eat. Her hypothalamus keeps track of just how much fat she has by constantly checking on her leptin level. When Susan became pregnant with Jessica her thirty-five pounds of fat produced nine units of leptin, but when David was conceived, she had forty-two pounds of fat and eleven units of leptin in her blood.

Because the amount of leptin in a woman's blood tells her hypothalamus how much stored body fat she has, it uses this as a guide for how much of the nutrients that come from her meals she should store and how much can circulate in her blood. When Susan digests a meal, insulin hormone sent out by her pancreas tells her cells to *save*. It tells her liver cells to save sugar, her fat cells to save fat, and her muscle cells to save amino acids and sugar. But when a woman already has plenty of fat, her hypothalamus tells her cells to pay less attention to her insulin's request to save. The more stored fat she has and the higher her leptin level, the more fat, sugar, and amino acids her hypothalamus allows her to keep in her blood. And if a woman has more stored fat when she becomes pregnant, she will have higher levels of these nutrients in her blood right from the start.

But depending on how much fat she has stored, these levels can go much higher during her pregnancy. When Susan became pregnant with Jessica and David and they began to grow in her womb, they each used their placentas to send Susan a hormonal message asking her to put even more sugar, fat, and amino acids into her blood as well as more DHA for their growing brains. And the more fat and leptin Susan has, the more willing her hypothalamus is to agree to their requests for more nutrients. With Jessica, Susan had enough fat to allow Jessica to grow to seven pounds. But when David came along, because of her added fat and higher leptin, Susan already had more sugar and fat in her blood, and she was even more willing to agree to his request for extra nutrients. Just as we are willing to spend more money on our children when we have more money in the bank, Susan's hypothalamus is willing to spend more of her stored fat on her babies when she has more in her fat account.

Because Susan has plenty of fat, her hypothalamus is also willing to let her blood pressure go up by a modest amount in order to help her baby grow more. Even though Susan releases extra nutrients into her bloodstream, the amount her baby gets also depends on how much of Susan's blood flows into the blood vessels in her womb where the placenta is attached and nutrients pass from her blood to her baby's. The amount of blood that goes to her womb depends on her blood pressure. Since Susan has plenty of fat and leptin, her hypothalamus allows her blood pressure to go a little higher so that more of her blood comes into contact with the placenta.

So a mother who has more of that unpopular waist fat helps her babies to grow more by putting larger amounts of critical nutrients into her bloodstream and pushing them toward the placenta with a higher blood pressure. As an added benefit, having more waist fat also increases the activity of Susan's white blood cells, which helps her to fight off any infections that threaten her and her baby during her pregnancy or while she is recovering from labor and nursing—times when women are more vulnerable to infection.

How much fat a mother like Susan has when she becomes pregnant has much more effect on how much her baby will weigh than her own genes do. When a woman becomes pregnant by using an egg cell donated by another woman, the birth weight of the baby is determined by the weight of the woman who receives the egg and carries the pregnancy, not by the weight of the woman who donated the egg.

Now we can better understand how and why Susan and Yasmin respond so differently during their pregnancies. In Susan's world, food is cheap and abundant. As a result, she is tall enough and has enough stored fat to be able to have a fairly large first child, Jessica. And afterward she can easily afford to put on the added fat that allows her to have an even bigger second child, David. Her hypothalamus allows her to spend more when she has more fat, and it encourages her to continue to add to her fat during her reproductive years so that she can afford to have larger children.

In contrast, Yasmin's lifelong struggle to get enough food has left her with much less in her fat account. So her hypothalamus is naturally very stingy and reluctant to part with much of her limited resources. It is much less responsive to the requests that come from Jemelah and Amir asking for more sugar, fat, amino acids, and DHA and for higher blood pressure. Yasmin cannot afford to give as generously as Susan, because she has to hold on to more of her limited fat just to stay alive and have the chance to give birth to other children. This keeps Jemelah and Amir from growing as much but also makes them better suited to a world in which food is scarce. In this way, the hypothalamus uses a mother's fat stores as a guide to keeping her children's size in balance with the amount of food that is available to her.

Women's bodies have a great deal of built-in wisdom. The *reason* a woman's weight and waist fat are linked to the amount of sugar, triglycerides, and amino acids in her blood and to her blood pressure is that these are what her babies need to grow. The more she weighs and the more fat she has, the more of these essential ingredients she makes available to help her babies grow bigger. Women who weigh more are not only likely to have bigger and healthier children, but also tend to have a larger number of children, which are both powerful reasons why genes for gaining weight when food is available are likely to be passed down from one generation of women to another.

So when more food is available, as it is for most American women today, women like Susan *need* to gain weight and add to their waist fat in order to give their children all the advantages that come from having a better food supply. A mother with more fat can afford to spend more of it on her children. She can afford to be heavier for her first child— but not so heavy that her baby will be too big to be born—and even heavier for her other children in order to prepare them to take full advantage of the world they will be living in. If she stayed thin, like Yasmin, her babies would grow less, have a harder time surviving infancy and childhood, and be at a disadvantage throughout their lives compared with the children whose mothers gained weight. Smaller sons would have a harder time winning the best mothers for their children; smaller daughters would have more difficulties with their own pregnancies. So even though a woman might wish she could stay as thin as she was in her late teens, her body *needs* her to gain more weight when enough food is available for the sake of her children.

What a Larger Waist Signals to Men

We have already uncovered two reasons why smaller waists are more attractive to men: Waist fat has less of the omega-3 fat needed for babies' brains, and it puts first-time mothers at greater risk of having a baby that is too big. But now we can add two other related reasons: Waist fat also indicates whether a woman has ever been pregnant and it helps reveal her age.

Since a woman tends to add more fat to her waist after giving birth, men can use a woman's waist size as a sign of whether or not she has been pregnant. A larger waist suggests that she has had a child and has used up some of her brain-building supplies and may also have another man's child to take care of; and the larger it is, the more children she is likely to have had. The smaller her waist size, the lower the chance that she has been pregnant before. Women with Playmate-size waists are very unlikely to have ever been pregnant. And as a woman continues to gain weight during her childbearing years, her waist size continues to grow; so the bigger her waist, the more children she is likely to have and the older she is likely to be.

But why should this be important to a young man? Though he is not aware of it, his selfish adaptive unconscious wants all of a young woman's resources and maternal attention for his children. A younger woman whose small waist says that she has not been pregnant before will be able to have more of his children. But if she already has a child, his children will have to compete for her attention and resources with her older children and, possibly, with the father of those children. And because a woman's capacity to have children has limits, each year that goes by means that she has less childbearing potential.

So these are added unconscious reasons why men find larger waists less attractive. In addition to storing less omega-3 and putting first-time mothers at risk for having babies that are too big to be born naturally, a bigger waist shows that a woman is likely to have already had a child and may be older. And because waists enlarge at the same time that some of the fat in the hips and legs is used up supplying precious omega-3 for the brain, this makes the waist-hip ratio an even stronger signal of a woman's potential value as a mother. Men have no idea why they have these preferences, but they help point the way to understanding why fat helps women to succeed in having children. Following these signposts helped us to better understand the wisdom of women's bodies and why they need fat.

When Placentas Attack

As Linda, a friend of Marcie and Ellen, was beginning the eighth month of her first pregnancy, she noticed that her hands and face seemed to be a bit puffy and that her ankles were more swollen than they had been. When she began her pregnancy, Linda was twenty-five pounds heavier than Marcie, weighing 175 pounds with a BMI of 30, the beginning of the "obese" range. Although she assumed that her puffiness was just another price you pay for being eight months pregnant, along with an aching back and an impatient bladder, she mentioned it to her obstetrician at her next prenatal visit. After examining her, the doctor told Linda that her blood pressure was now elevated above the normal range and that she also had some protein in her urine; this meant that her swelling was due to a condition called *preeclampsia*. Fortunately, her obstetrician was able to keep Linda's blood pressure from going much higher and solved her problem by delivering a healthy but small baby boy, Ethan, four weeks later.

Preeclampsia is twice as likely to happen during a first pregnancy, and it affects one in sixteen first-time American mothers. Heavier mothers like Linda are much more likely to develop it. So avoiding this condition is yet another reason why it's helpful for a mother to be thinner for her first pregnancy. But why is preeclampsia more likely to strike heavier first-time mothers like Linda?

We just saw that a healthy placenta produces hormones that ask the mother to increase her blood pressure by a modest amount. Heavier women are more responsive to this request, and this can help them to have bigger babies by bringing more blood to the placenta. But their blood pressure usually still stays well within the normal range. But Linda's blood pressure went much higher than what would be normal for a heavier mother, because her baby's placenta was in a state of panic and was sending out torrents of hormones to drive up Linda's pressure.

Linda's placenta was pouring out hormones because her son Ethan was having difficulty getting enough oxygen and nutrients from his placenta. In order to provide enough oxygen and nutrients for a big-brained baby to grow well, the cells of the placenta have to burrow very deeply into the wall of the womb to where the bigger arteries are located. But since half of Ethan's genes come from his father Jerry, Linda's white blood cells—more active because of her higher weight—regarded these burrowing cells as foreign invaders and responded by making antibodies to repel them. This is much more likely to happen during a first pregnancy because Linda's white cells are not yet well acquainted with Jerry's genes. By the time Linda's next child comes along, they will be more friendly. Heavier mothers like Linda are more likely to have this problem because their extra waist fat makes their white blood cells more active and more likely to attack the placental cells. So just like obstructed labor, this problem is strongly linked to a mother's weight before her pregnancy. A very thin first-time mother like Ellen has less than a 3 percent chance of developing preeclampsia, while a heavier mother like Marcie has a 15 percent chance, and an obese mother like Linda, a 30 percent chance.

Linda was fortunate to have medical assistance, but if a mother's blood pressure cannot be controlled, she may go into convulsions and even die. Despite modern blood pressure drugs and the ability to deliver babies early, four first-time American mothers in a thousand still develop serious convulsions due to preeclampsia; and this is a major cause of death during pregnancy in the United States. This is bad enough, but without medical treatment, it is a much more serious problem in developing countries and causes the deaths of many more mothers. So in addition to the perils of obstructed labor, this is another important reason why it is beneficial for a first-time mother to be fairly thin and for men to admire narrow waists.

Too Much of a Good Thing? Obesity and Pregnancy

Before the unfortunate dietary changes of the last few decades, most American women gained enough weight to reach the overweight category during their childbearing years, but very few became obese. In the 1960s, fewer than one in seventeen women in her twenties was obese, and for women in their thirties, it was fewer than one in seven. In contrast, today more than a third of American women of childbearing age gain enough weight to become "obese," like Linda. And as Linda's problem with preeclampsia shows, obese mothers are more likely to have certain problems during pregnancy and labor that would have been a great disadvantage before modern medical care.

As a mother's weight increases, the amount of sugar in her blood can rise so high that she develops a temporary form of diabetes. This happens to about one in fifteen obese mothers and is three times more likely for them than for women who weigh less. Because of the high levels of sugar and fat in their blood, their babies tend to grow very large, and this can be hazardous for both mother and child. Half of obese mothers require a surgical delivery, and very big babies are more likely to have serious problems before and after birth. Because today's teens are already much heavier than their mothers were as teens, these pregnancy-related problems are likely to increase as they begin having children of their own. Fortunately, most obese mothers and their babies still do well when they have ready access to good medical care from the start of their pregnancies. But before modern medical care, obese mothers would have been at a big disadvantage. Having early and regular prenatal care is especially important for heavier mothers.

How Does a Woman's Brain Make Her Gain Weight?

Almost all women gain weight after having a child because this benefits her subsequent children. But just how is this managed? What actually causes them to gain weight? Once again, it's our body's building supervisor, the hypothalamus, at work. In addition to its role in deciding when a woman can start her periods and how much a mother can give to her baby during her pregnancy, it also controls our weight.

Although it might not seem like it, our hypothalamus usually keeps our weights within very narrow limits, matching our intake of calories very precisely to how much we spend—much better than we could ever do if we tried to keep track consciously. If we ask adult Americans—men and women—how much they weighed one year ago and how much they weigh today, almost four in ten weigh exactly the same; and the typical change in weight is very small for most of the others. It seems that our brain has a target weight for each of us that it strives to maintain, what has been called the "set point" for our weights.

When Susan was in her teens, her hypothalamus encouraged her to store a total of thirty-five pounds of fat, enough to bring the leptin level in her blood up to nine units, and that was her "set point." It kept it at this level by making her hungrier when it dropped below nine and less hungry if it went above. After Jessica was born (and her body knew she would have plenty to eat), Susan's hypothalamus allowed her leptin level to rise to eleven, which in turn made her heavier for her next pregnancy—so she could support a bigger second baby. And so that any later babies she might have could be heavier and healthier, it allowed her leptin to continue to rise. Before American weights started going up, Susan's brain would have let her leptin level slowly increase so that she would gain weight until she reached a leptin level of around eighteen, which would have allowed her weight to go up to 145 to 150 pounds sometime in her forties. The hypothalamus encourages women to gain this weight after having a child so that they can have healthier children in the future. But today, because of the unnatural changes in the American diet, our brains are allowing much higher limits on our leptin levels and higher "set points." In Susan's case, for example, her brain has let her leptin level soar to twenty-two, and she has gained much more weight as a result.

It may be surprising to know that when women like Susan gain weight, it's not because they're eating tons of extra calories. A weight gain of one pound a year amounts to just nine extra calories a day, an amount so small that you cannot measure it by weighing food. Even with today's "obesity epidemic," the average gain of one and a half pounds a year amounts to a mere fourteen extra calories a day. So even when we gain, our brain still keeps our food intake within remarkably tight limits.

Why Do Women Who Have Not Had Children Gain Weight?

We have seen that while a woman benefits by adding fat after her first child is born, it is better for her to weigh less before her first pregnancy to lower her risk of having a baby that is too big or having blood pressure problems. Thus, until recently, a woman without children usually did not gain much weight in her twenties and early thirties. But as she gets older, even a childless woman may also begin to gain weight. This seems to run counter to the idea that women's bodies keep them relatively thin until they have a child. Why should her age matter?

When a woman gets into her thirties without having a child, she has less time left on her "biological clock" for having children. Though modern fertility treatments can help, her chances of becoming pregnant and having a healthy baby go down with each passing year. From the viewpoint of her genes, time is running out for them to make it into the next generation. Because the stakes are getting higher, her selfish genes are willing for her to take more risks. For a twenty-year-old woman without children, it is better to be safe than sorry, since she is likely to have other chances to have a child; so her genes try to keep her thin. Her first child may be smaller and more vulnerable, but she has plenty of time to have more children. But the trade-offs are different for an older woman with no children. Although gaining weight increases her risk of a difficult delivery and blood pressure problems, it also makes it more likely that any baby that does make it through her birth canal will be a strong and healthy one. So while this is not something she consciously decides, her genes may be willing to take the bet that her being heavier will give her baby a better chance to survive and so may push her to gain more weight. Women in their early thirties who have not had children usually continue to maintain lower weights; but after age thirty-four, weights typically begin to increase by one to two pounds a year—a faster rate than for women this age who have had children—and by their late forties, they have often caught up with the moms.

We can see actual signs of this greater risk-taking if we look at what happens to women who have their first pregnancy after their midthirties, when many have begun to gain weight. Their risk of having a first baby that is too big are more than twice as high as they are for younger first-time mothers, and their risk of having preeclampsia is one-third higher.

Although women who do not have children may catch up in weight to those who do, women who have their first child at a later age than average usually tend to gain less weight than women who have their first child earlier. Many American women today are choosing to wait until they are older before they have a child. Of those mothers who gave birth for the first time in 1990, two-thirds were under the age of twenty-five compared with just half in 2008. But unlike most of our recent dietary changes, delaying a first pregnancy can actually help women keep weight off.

For women under thirty-five, weights tend to stay relatively low before they have their first child, and then start to go up after they have a baby. This means that women who are younger when they have their first child start gaining weight earlier and have more time to gain weight during their childbearing years. For this reason, teenage mothers tend to gain the most weight. As a result, until recently, women who have their first child later than average weigh less in their forties than women with earlier first births. But unfortunately, because our unnatural diets today are causing many young women without children to gain much more weight than they did in the past, any advantage that they might gain by delaying childbirth is likely to be overwhelmed by these unfortunate dietary effects.

Why Women Need Fat

We have now answered our questions about why women's fat is so unusual and why men pay so much attention to it. A girl stores fat throughout her childhood in her legs and hips to bank the omega-3 DHA that her children will need in order to have a large and well-functioning brain. But her waist fat remains limited, to lower her chances of having a first baby that is too big to be born or of developing preeclampsia. Gaining weight after having her first baby is beneficial for any other babies that follow. So if she has food available, she *needs* to gain more weight so that her children will be able to take full advantage of living in a world where food is plentiful.

Men find the fat in a woman's hips, legs, and buttocks attractive because it holds an omega-3 treasure trove, while waist fat has less omega-3, endangers a first-time mother, and suggests that a woman has already had a child and is older. Since both smaller waists and fatter hips are desirable for first-time mothers and because both make the waist-hip ratio smaller, this explains why low waist-hip ratios are so universally attractive to men.

The Link Between a Woman's Natural Weight Gain and Today's Higher Weights

While this normal pattern of weight gain is encoded in our genes and has been the same for well-fed women over thousands of years, we are now seeing something quite new and unexpected. Because of the unnatural changes in the American diet, younger American women are much heavier now than they have ever been in the past, and women with children have been gaining much more weight after they give birth.

One reason American women are heavier today than in the past is related to their natural need for fat. For many thousands of years, young women have stored DHA in their lower-body fat to provide for their children while remaining relatively thin. But this natural pattern evolved in an environment where there was more valuable omega-3 fats than the competing omega-6 fats—where a smaller amount of omega-3s was not being swamped by a tsunami of industrially produced omega-6s. The high level of omega-3 and modest amount of omega-6 in their diets allowed them to store enough DHA without needing to be very heavy, just as is true for women with diets high in omega-3 and low in omega-6 today, like the Japanese.

The situation for American women today is very different and quite unprecedented, because their omega fats are so severely out of balance. Although we have a seeming abundance of food, our very unnatural diet is extremely high in omega-6 fat and quite low in omega-3 fat, especially the longer forms of omega-3—DHA and EPA—that our brains and bodies require. The exceedingly high levels of omega-6 make it much more difficult for women to store and convert omega-3 and to have sufficient DHA and EPA—the fats that lower weights.

Because of this unnatural omega balance, American women now have much less DHA in their blood and a much lower percentage of DHA in their fat than they would have had in the past. The only way they can have a total DHA level closer to women with a diet with a more natural balance in omega-3 is by storing more fat. And this applies not only to women before their first pregnancy but also to women who have had children. Since each pregnancy and nursing period draws down on a mother's supply of DHA, gaining weight after having a child helps to restore some of the DHA that she has lost. Although much of the new weight she gains goes to her waist, some also goes to her lower body and contains additional DHA. But when a mother has low levels of DHA in her blood, her hypothalamus may push her to gain even more weight after having a child to help restore some of the DHA that she has lost from her more limited supply.

Since most of the DHA in a woman's milk comes from her stored fat, we can get an idea of the percentage of DHA in a woman's fat from the amount of DHA she has in her milk. In Japanese women, for example—a group with high omega-3, low omega-6, and very low rates of obesity—about 1 percent of their milk fat is DHA. This is *six times* as much as in the milk of American mothers, who have nearly the lowest percentage of DHA in the world.

Because American women have such low levels of DHA, the only way they can store more DHA is by adding more fat. This helps to explain why the average American woman weighs *forty* pounds more than the average woman in Japan with the same height, why obesity is twenty-seven times more common in American women, and why they are storing much more fat than their mothers and grandmothers did at their age. A natural diet leads to a natural amount of stored fat; an unnatural diet leads to excess fat. In the next part of the book, we will look at what women can do to try to reverse these changes and move back to their natural, healthy weight.

Part Three

How to Achieve Your
Healthy Natural Weight

CHAPTER 6

Myths About Weight and Health

A s her doctor knocks gently, the moment Susan has been dreading has arrived. Once again, she'll have to hear why her extra pounds are bad for her. If only her doctor weren't quite so informative. Sure enough, he tells her that her BMI puts her in the high end of the overweight category and explains that her extra fat can increase her blood sugar, triglycerides, blood pressure, and white blood cell activity, and lower her good cholesterol, or HDL. And these consequences of being overweight may increase her risk of heart disease, stroke, and diabetes.

This is disturbing news; but haven't we just seen that gaining weight during childbearing years is natural and beneficial for women? Isn't having higher sugar, triglycerides, and blood pressure exactly what helps mothers like Susan to have heavier, healthier babies? Has Mother Nature played a nasty trick on women? Does gaining weight help women to have healthier babies at the cost of making them sick? These are complex questions, but when we cut through the mythology and prejudice we find that they have remarkable and unexpected answers.

The Rumors of Our Deaths Have Been
Greatly Exaggerated

Dr. Katherine Flegal was perplexed. It was a pleasant March day in Atlanta in 2004, and she was reading a brand-new journal article titled "Actual Causes of Death in the United States." One of the authors, Dr. Julie Gerberding, was Katherine's top boss as the director of the Centers for Disease Control and Prevention, the federal agency where Katherine had worked for the past eighteen years. In the article, Gerberding and three other CDC scientists claimed that being overweight or obese is responsible for more than four hundred thousand American deaths a year—one of every five—and that excess weight would soon surpass tobacco use as our number one preventable cause of death.

That evening, Gerberding appeared on national television to emphasize her message that obesity is a killer. In a segment called "Americans Eat Themselves to Death" for CBS News, she proclaimed that "our worst fears have been confirmed," and added, "At CDC, we're going to do everything we can to prevent it. Obesity has got to be job number one for us in terms of chronic diseases." She was quoted in *USA Today* saying that the study's results were a "tragedy" and told the *Washington Post* that "we're looking at this as a wake-up call," while her boss, Secretary of Health and Human Services Tommy Thompson, added, "Americans need to understand that overweight and obesity are literally killing us."

Gerberding clearly had strong opinions on the dangers of higher weights. A few months earlier, she had compared the consequences of the American obesity epidemic to the ravages of the Black Death—the epidemic of plague that killed some 75 million Europeans in the 1300s (half the population at the time)—and to the influenza epidemic of 1919 that killed 50 million people. She had said, "If you look at any epidemic—whether it's influenza or plague from the Middle Ages—they are not as serious as the epidemic of obesity in terms of the health impact on our country and our society." She was pulling out all the stops to convince Americans that obesity was very bad news for their health.

But none of this made sense to Dr. Flegal, the CDC scientist in charge of tracking weight and obesity in the United States. Flegal was certain that Gerberding's one-death-in-five claim was wrong. And she quickly realized that the method Gerberding had used to estimate the number of deaths caused by higher weights was the same faulty approach used in an earlier study claiming that obesity was causing large numbers of deaths. Flegal and two of her colleagues had just written a paper showing that this method was badly flawed and greatly exaggerated the harmful effects of higher weight. They were also already well along on their own carefully designed study of the effect of weight on the health of Americans based on three large-scale national surveys.

What Flegal's team found in their study was quite different from what her boss was proclaiming: Death rates were *higher* in those who were thin, *lowest* in those who were overweight (with a BMI of 25 to 29), and only a little higher in those with "mild" obesity (a BMI of 30 to 35), which includes fully half of the American women classified as obese. They found that rather than four hundred thousand deaths a year from being overweight or obese as Gerberding claimed, there were fewer than thirteen thousand, or just one death in 180—much lower than Gerberding's one in five. Flegal's group also found that the more recent the study, the better the survival of those who were heavier. In other words, as more Americans were getting heavier, the health risks of being heavy seemed to be diminishing.

After her team's own results were published, Flegal was quite surprised when they were passionately attacked by other obesity researchers. Many experts in assessing health risks had reviewed her study and judged it to be very well designed and executed, and she had thought people would be glad to hear that being overweight or obese was not so bad. But some leading obesity researchers urged their colleagues to contact their local media to counter Flegal's message in order to help ensure continued funding for their research and assure a steady flow of overweight patients for their clinics.

The most egregious attack came from obesity researchers at Harvard. Instead of trying to use scientific methods to show that Flegal's team had made mistakes, they commissioned a public opinion poll. They were quite pleased to report that most Americans were still quite convinced that being overweight or obese poses a grave danger to health and that four out of five considered it to be "very" or "extremely" serious. Half of the people surveyed believed that more people die from being "overweight" than from smoking. Of course, public opinions have nothing to do with whether Flegal was right.

In fact, most of her critics did not dispute the validity of her study; instead they backpedaled and denied claiming that excess weight was causing many unnecessary deaths. Said one, "I do not believe that the scientific community has promoted mortality as the big reason that obesity is such a serious public health threat." He seemed to have forgotten the comparison of obesity with the Black Death. Meanwhile, an internal investigation by the CDC requested by a congressman determined that Gerberding's estimate was indeed wrong. She later held a press conference to apologize and affirm the validity of Flegal's study, but then contradicted herself by asserting, "It is not okay to be overweight."

Most of the criticism of Dr. Flegal's study had come from obesity researchers whose livelihoods depend on the public believing that obesity is bad for health. Many of these researchers have strong ties to companies that make weight-loss products. David Allison, lead author of the study used as the model for Gerberding's, acknowledged that he had received grants, money, and products from "numerous organizations selling weight control products and services." Selling such products and services to American women is a $40-billion-a-year industry; an industry that depends, at least in part, on the idea that being obese is a terrible thing.

The Truth About Obesity and Being Overweight

If the campaign to magnify the health risks of being overweight or obese is beginning to remind you of Keys's campaign against fat, you're right; they are quite similar. Just as there are no studies showing that changing your diet helps you to live longer, *there are no studies showing that overweight or obese women who lose weight live longer.* In fact, the studies of those who lose weight, including those who lose weight on purpose, show that they tend to die sooner, not later.

Flegal's study was by no means the first to find that being overweight (with a BMI of 25 to 29) seems to actually be healthy for women. There have been more than sixty medical studies that have looked at the health effects of being overweight in women over forty. Far from showing a higher death rate from being overweight, most of these studies agree with Flegal's findings and show that overweight women like Susan tend to live longer than women with lower weights. The few studies that show lower survival in overweight women have serious problems with their methods. So the same "overweight" group that many women naturally move into after they have children is also the group with the best health.

Again like Flegal's, many other studies also show that women with "mild obesity" (a BMI of 30 to 34) tend to have similar life spans to women with lower weights. While some studies show a small decrease in life span, many show no survival difference between mildly obese and overweight women, and some even show that survival is highest in this group (especially in older women).

For women with still higher weights, however, obesity does seem to be less healthy and to reduce life span. For those with a BMI of 35 to 39 (204 to 232 pounds), there is an average loss of about three years of life, and for those who are heavier (BMIs of 40 and above), a loss of about eight years is typical. Having many more women in this group of very high BMIs may be one reason why American women rank thirtieth in the world in life expectancy. They live about two years less on average than women in twenty-nine countries—all places where obesity rates are much lower.

One reason that obese women may be less healthy is that one in five develops diabetes. Another is that they tend to be less active than women with lower weights—walking less, for example—and only half as likely to engage in vigorous exercise. Obese women who are physically active have much better survival rates than those who are sedentary. Also, some of the same genetic combinations that lead to very high weights may also have other adverse health effects unconnected with weight. Finally, the higher omega-6 and lower omega-3 levels linked with heavier weights may also undermine their health. So while a high-omega-3/low-omega-6 diet has been shown to be good for the health of all women, it may be particularly beneficial for heavier women.

Most of the researchers who attacked Flegal's study conceded that being overweight or "mildly" obese does not greatly decrease life span, yet they were the same ones who had been promoting the very high estimates of deaths due to being overweight or obese that make people think excess weight is very unhealthy. Because many Americans are biased against heavier women—including many women who are them-selves overweight or obese—they are predisposed to believe that any excess weight must be very bad for health and that heavier women must die earlier, as the Harvard public opinion poll shows.

There is also one other reason why physicians may tend to overes-timate the dangers of obesity, especially physicians who are older: Obesity used to be less healthy than it is today. Before the 1970s, American women usually weighed much less than they do now and obesity was much less common, but, because of their genes, some women—one in seven or eight—were still obese. They were obese because they happened to fall into the small percentage of women who inevitably inherit a set of genes that makes them very likely to be quite heavy if they have enough to eat.

But as Dr. Flegal's research suggests, the obese women of fifty years ago seem to have been less healthy than obese women today. The gene combinations that caused their higher weights may have had other negative effects on their health separate from their effect on their weights. Today, the relatively small percentage of women with this same obesity-promoting set of genes tend to be much heavier than in the past, usually weighing more than 225 pounds, and they are still at high risk for poor health. But a majority of women who are obese today would not have been obese were they still eating the American diet of the 1960s, before the flood of omega-6s. They are obese only because of the unnatural American diet they are now eating. Because they do not have the same unhealthy combination of genes that made women obese in the past, they are healthier than those women were. But those physicians who did their training before the current obesity epidemic may still be basing their judgments on their experience with patients from that era or on earlier medical studies.

Fat Protects Women from Serious Infections

We have seen that being overweight has health advantages for American women today, but being overweight or even obese also has an even greater health benefit that is difficult for Americans to fully appreciate: resistance to infection. Because of antibiotics and an abundance of food, infections are much less of a threat to the health of Americans now than they were in the past, despite our recent epidemic of HIV/AIDS. Infections now account for less than one death in ten, and most of those are in the elderly. But when diseases caused by infection are a serious problem, as they have been for most of human history, the health advantages of being overweight are even stronger. In Bangladesh, for instance, where women are much thinner, one death in four is due to infection, though other factors are also involved.

Just 150 years ago, one of every two American deaths was due to infection; for example, the leading cause of death was the lung infection tuberculosis. Overweight and obese women were much less vulnerable to these serious infections than thinner women. The heavier a woman was, the less likely she was to get or die from tuberculosis, while thinner women were much more vulnerable. The stories of that era, like *Camille*, tell of many slender young women succumbing to this dreaded disease. Many medical studies show that women with lower weights are the most likely to die from infections.

Heavier women are less vulnerable to serious infections like tuberculosis because they have more active white blood cells. Compared with men, all women have more active infection-fighting cells and more of them. Because women have more fat than men (and less testosterone), they have larger numbers of more active white blood cells and more of the immune factors they produce in their blood; and their death rate from infections is one-third lower than men's. Doctors often assess white cell activity by measuring C-reactive protein (CRP) in the blood and warn patients with high levels that they may be at greater risk for blood vessel diseases. But women naturally have higher CRP levels than men and still have a much lower risk of blood vessel diseases, and heavier women have even higher levels. More active white cells give better protection from the infections that have taken the most young lives during human history; and they especially help women survive pregnancy and childbirth, which both increase their risk of infection. And, as we will see now, Mother Nature has also protected women from the potentially harmful effects of having more active immune cells. So having more fat in times and parts of the world with high infection rates has even greater health advantages for women.

Why Being Overweight *Ought* to Be Bad for Women

To be fair, there are reasons why physicians would *expect* higher weights in women to be unhealthy. It isn't just a conspiracy between obesity researchers and the weight-loss industry. These reasons involve what physicians call "risk factors" for disease. Every day they see that their heavier patients, like Susan, tend to have higher levels of blood pressure, triglycerides, blood sugar, and white blood cell activity (like CRP), and lower levels of HDL. Each of these is a risk factor for coronary disease, even though (except for HDL) they help women to have healthier babies.

Because heavier *men* with these "risk factors" are more likely to develop coronary disease at a younger age, it is natural to think that they should be bad for women's health as well. But evolution has strongly linked these factors to women's weights because they help women have better babies. Women need to gain weight when they can—but not at the expense of their health and survival. Mothers must survive for their babies to thrive. So how does nature strike a balance that allows for healthier babies and a healthy mother?

Estrogen Explains Why Being Overweight *Isn't* Bad for Women

The main way that nature protects a mother from the unhealthy effects of being overweight is with her estrogen hormone. While a woman's higher levels of blood sugar, triglyceride, blood pressure, and white blood cell activity ought to be making her arteries thicken, they don't because her estrogen blocks their effects on her blood vessels. During the Korean War, army doctors were surprised to find that many young American soldiers already had fatty deposits almost blocking some of their coronary arteries. But because of women's estrogen hormone, most women don't begin this process until much later in their lives, usually after their periods stop and their estrogen production falls.

Estrogen also gives women much more of the good cholesterol—HDL—than men, as well as higher levels of heart-healthy omega-3 in their blood. And while HDL is a little lower in heavier American women, it is still higher than in men. It may go down in heavier women because they exercise less, drink less alcohol, and have higher amounts of soybean and corn oil in their diet—all things that lower HDL. Because of estrogen's great protective power, women have been *seven times* less likely than men to die of·coronary disease before age sixty-five (though smoking cuts this benefit in half).

In addition to the estrogen made by their ovaries, heavier women also make more estrogen out of the male hormone testosterone. All women produce some testosterone in their adrenal glands and ovaries, and fat cells can convert this testosterone into estrogen. Because heavier women have more fat cells, they convert more of their natural testosterone to estrogen than thinner women do. This helps them to have a later and easier menopause than lighter women, extending their period of maximum protection from blood vessel disease. So nature has designed women to get fatter after their first baby, but it has also given them very strong protection from any harmful effects of gaining that weight.

While estrogen has great benefits for women's health, there is sometimes an unfortunate downside to having more estrogen. Although it delays the blood vessel changes that cause heart attacks and strokes, it can also stimulate the estrogen-sensitive cells in a woman's breasts. Curiously, women who are heavier in their teens have *less* chance of developing breast cancer later in life, and women who are heavier when they are older are also *less* likely to have breast cancer *before* age fifty. However, middle-aged obese women are a little more likely to have breast cancer after age fifty. Overall, one in nine American women develop breast cancer after age fifty, and one in thirty-seven die from it. Most women in the "overweight" range of BMIs do not have increased risk. But studies suggest that for obese women, the risk of developing breast cancer after fifty increases by a fourth, to one in seven, and the chance of dying from this cancer rises to one in thirty.

Because of this increased risk, having regular mammograms and breast exams is especially important for heavier women. In addition, studies have shown that omega-3 fats reduce the chances of breast cancer while omega-6 fats increase the risk, so it is even more important for heavier women to follow our recommendations for increasing omega-3 and decreasing omega-6 in their diets to reduce their chances of developing breast cancer as well as helping to lower their weights.

Despite their extra estrogen, overweight and obese women are also still much more likely to develop diabetes than women with lower weights. The heavier a woman is, the more insulin the cells in her pancreas have to make each day, and over time, these cells can wear out. One in twelve overweight women develops diabetes, twice as many as women with lower weights. This increases to one in eight with mild obesity and to one in four for still heavier women. Over the past twenty years, although American women have been living longer, their death rate from diabetes has increased by a third. Losing weight may benefit heavier women with diabetes by lowering their blood sugar levels. Fortunately, a high-omega-3/low-omega-6 diet can also help to prevent diabetes by lowering blood sugar, yet another way that changing to this kind of diet is especially beneficial for heavier women.

Bones, Joints, and Weight:
Bad News, Good News

For bones and joints, being heavier is a mixed blessing. Because heavier women put more stress on the hip, knee, spine, and ankle joints that support their weight, this increases their chances of developing arthritis in those joints. Being in the "overweight" range does not have much effect on the joints, but obese women have double the risk and one in four develop arthritis. These joint problems are the most common adverse health effects of high weights and are the problems most likely to make heavier women feel unhealthy and to interfere with their ability to work or exercise.

But even though being heavier can increase the likelihood of arthritis, there is also an upside for heavier women. Because there is more stress on their bones, they become stronger and thicker. In addition, heavier women's fat cells also give them more bone-building estrogen. As a result, they tend to lose less calcium from the bones in their legs and spine (and arms) as they age and to be much less likely to have broken bones in later life. Overall, one in five American women will suffer a broken hip, and this often leads to a downward spiral, with a quarter of the women who have had a hip fracture dying within a year of the injury. Because heavier women's increased weight strengthens their leg and hip bones, they are less likely to break their hips. Women with the highest weights have just one-third the hip-fracture risk of women with the lowest weights. This beneficial effect of weight on bone strength is about twice as great as the effect of regular exercise.

So there is a kind of compensation: The more arthritis a woman has, the less likely she will be to have a hip fracture. Being heavier also makes the bones in her spine stronger, so that a heavier woman is less likely to have collapse of her vertebral bones and shortening of her neck and spine. A recent study has found that *not* losing weight and having strong bones are the two most important things in determining how long older women live and how healthy they feel. So while being heavier can stress joints, it also has significant benefits.

Good Fat, Bad Fat: Is Waist Size More Important than Weight?

In addition to the effect of your weight on your health, the location of your fat may also be important. As American women have been getting heavier, their waist sizes have been increasing even more rapidly than their weight. This is important because many studies have shown that women with more waist fat have a higher risk for diabetes, heart disease, and other health problems, while lower-body fat seems to be healthier—as Dev Singh learned from his doctor. Just as waist fat has a stronger effect on birth weights, all of the "risk factors" linked to weight are more strongly related to the amount of waist fat than to weight itself. Though waist fat naturally increases as weight goes up, some studies have found that waist size is more important than weight alone in predicting survival and health. Women with more waist fat tend to have less health-promoting omega-3 DHA, while those with more lower-body fat (hip and thigh fat) and a lower waist-hip ratio tend to have more omega-3 and to be healthier. Women with a waist size over thirty-five inches measured just above the hips (the "trouser waist") seem to be at a greater risk for poor health.

In just the last fifteen years, the average waist size for American women with the same BMI has increased by almost an inch (probably due to our increased consumption of vegetable oils). In the early 1990s, about half of women in the overweight group had waist sizes in the unhealthy over-thirty-five-inch range, but today roughly three out of four do. And one in seven women with "normal" weights now also have unhealthy waist sizes. These larger waist sizes may be contributing to the recent increase in the number of women with diabetes, and it is possible that they will also have other effects on their health as women get older. These are yet more reasons to make a change and eat a more natural diet to lower your weight and your waist size.

What About Young Women Who Are Overweight or Obese?

As we saw earlier, weights have been increasing even more dramatically in young American women—like Susan's daughter Jessica. Forty years ago, one in six young women was overweight; today, nearly half are overweight, and one in four is obese. Assuming that they continue to gain weight as they age in the same way as their mothers, two-thirds will become obese by middle age.

It is difficult to predict what effect this extra weight will have on the health of the heavier young women of today as they age. In the past, when being overweight was quite rare in young women, those who were overweight in their teens were likely to have poorer health later in life, and three out of four developed diabetes. But this does not necessarily tell us what will happen with the larger numbers of young women who are overweight or obese today, since recent studies, like Dr. Flegal's, suggest that heavier women are healthier today than they were in the past. It is likely, however, that many will develop diabetes from having more years of making extra insulin. And those whose BMIs climb past 40 will definitely be at greater risk for health problems.

Even though estrogen protects women from many of the harmful effects of being heavier, the likelihood of health problems like breast cancer, diabetes, and arthritis is still increased. So moving back toward the lower weights that young women have had in the past by changing to a more natural diet should be beneficial for the health of everyone, and the same diet may also help to counter some of the adverse health effects heavier women face.

Gaining Is Good (Up to a Point)

In order to provide a better chance for their later babies, women are genetically programmed to gain weight after they have a child; and they typically move from the "normal" to the "overweight" range as a result of this built-in weight-gain program. However, most studies show that becoming overweight does not make them less healthy; if anything, it makes them healthier. So nature has not punished women for doing what comes naturally.

However, as weights rise well into the "obese" range and move past two hundred pounds, there is often a decrease in health and life span; and having a baby also becomes more hazardous. Regular exercise and health care, and avoiding other risk factors for poor health—such as inactivity and cigarette smoking—is especially important for these heavier women. In addition, changing to the same high-omega-3/ low-omega-6 diet that can help women weigh less can also reduce their risk for poor health. For those who develop diabetes, losing some weight may also be beneficial. But a return to a more natural diet—one with a better balance of omega-3 and omega-6 fats—should help lower the weights and improve the health of all women.

CHAPTER 7

Why Dieting Doesn't Work

Susan's experience of dieting, losing weight, gaining it back, and ending up heavier than when she started is all too common in American women. Each year in the past decade, almost two out of every three American women report having tried to lose weight by dieting. Despite their repeated efforts to lose weight, the average dieter has *gained* fourteen pounds over those ten years, and one in three dieters has gained twenty-five pounds or more. Fewer than one in twenty weighs less than she did ten years ago, and even for these few the difference is very small. Never before have so many women spent so much money, expended so much effort, and endured so much suffering in so futile an effort.

It's not that American women aren't successful in losing weight; many are, in fact, prodigiously successful—for a time. In the past year, more than 60 million American women tried to lose weight. One in three—20 million women—ended the year weighing less, losing an average of sixteen pounds. Unfortunately, the evidence strongly suggests that almost all of them will regain the weight they lost—and more—just as those who lost weight in previous years have done. A larger number of the women who tried to lose—two out of five—finished the year already weighing *more*, gaining an average of fifteen pounds. Many of these women probably also lost weight at some point during the year but gained back even more. The rest of the women who tried to lose weight—one in four—ended up exactly where they started, though many of them may have also lost weight at some time during the year. Through rigid self-control and an extraordinary willingness to suffer, millions of American women succeed in losing weight each year, and yet most not only gain it all back but end up weighing more than when they started.

So how did young women stay so thin from the 1890s to the 1970s when average weights in American women were considerably lower and remarkably constant? Were they constantly dieting? Judging from the number of diet books and articles in magazines, that's not the reason. In the entire decade from 1950 to 1960, only five American books about dieting were published. Today, that many diet books are published in a typical week! So it seems that a half century ago, before Ancel Keys and the *Dietary Goals*, women didn't diet but still maintained much lower weights. Today most women diet but gain weight. This seems like a paradox. Could it be that dieting itself tends to increase weight?

Doing What Does Not Come Naturally

Jeffrey was one of thirty-six conscientious objectors during World War II who volunteered to live for a year at Ancel Keys's nutrition laboratory at the University of Minnesota to participate in a study of the effects of food deprivation. Keys knew that many European countries were already suffering food shortages and that these conditions would likely worsen as the Allies moved across France and into Germany. He wanted to better understand how a healthy body responds to a shortage of food.

The first step in the study was to see how many calories Jeffrey needed to maintain his current weight; this came to 3,400 calories per day. He was then cut back to half that level, 1,700 calories, a level similar to many weight-loss diets. He was also asked to walk three miles a day. During his first twelve weeks on this diet, he lost twenty pounds, but during his next twelve weeks on the same diet, he lost only nine pounds. As happens with most dieters, his weight loss slowed down even though he stuck to the same regimen.

As the weeks went by, Jeffrey became increasingly weak, lethargic, and apathetic. His pulse rate slowed, his metabolism fell by almost half, and he became totally obsessed with food. He got in line at the cafeteria an hour before mealtime, and he usually licked his plate clean of every crumb. He often took bits of the food he was given to his room and ate them in a ritual that could last for hours. The only thing he and the other volunteers talked about was food. He read only cookbooks and food magazines and talked incessantly about recipes with the other volunteers. He drank coffee and tea all day long and was finally limited to nine cups a day. He lost interest in sex. At the movies, he only wanted to watch scenes where people were eating. Five of his fellow volunteers could not make it through the six-month experiment. Two became suicidal; another broke into the kitchen and binged on food; and one was maniacally chewing forty packs of gum a day.

After six months on the low-calorie diet, Jeffrey was finally allowed to return to his normal intake of 3,400 calories for another ten weeks, but he still felt constantly and ravenously hungry and continued to be apathetic and depressed. Finally he was allowed to eat anything he wanted, and immediately he almost tripled the amount of food he ate each day, far above his normal intake. But even though he was stuffing himself, he still felt hungry all the time. After ten weeks eating whatever he wanted, he was fifteen pounds heavier than he had been at the beginning of the experiment and was still hungry. Dieting had made him fat.

Twenty years later, a team at Rockefeller University led by Dr. Jules Hirsch saw this same kind of behavior pattern in a group of very obese men and women after they had been on a very low-calorie diet for four months. Most had weighed more than three hundred pounds, and the average participant had lost more than eighty pounds during the diet phase. But even though they still had much more body fat than an average person, they behaved just like Keys's volunteers—like someone who is starving—and became completely obsessed with food.

Despite looking better and feeling quite pleased with their lower weights, they soon gained back all the weight they had lost, and many ended up heavier than when they began the program. This led Hirsch to the idea that each of us has a "set point" for our weight, a weight that our brains consider right for us. The brains of his dieters were determined to make their bodies go back at least to their original higher weights because these were their personal set points.

At about the same time, a few hundred miles to the north, Ethan Sims, a physician at the University of Vermont, was trying to see if he could make four typical college students get fat. He had been trying to make mice fat and found that it was surprisingly difficult. He started the students off on *twice* their usual number of calories. For example, one student, Winston Morris, who weighed 188 pounds, was given 6,700 calories a day! If our weight depended only on how many calories we eat, he should have been gaining almost a pound a day. But after two months of eating this enormous number of calories, Winston did not gain a single pound. So Sims upped his calories to 10,200 a day, *three times* his normal intake. After two months on this supersize diet, Winston finally did manage to gain some weight, but as soon as the experiment was over, those extra pounds quickly melted away and he was soon back to his previous weight. Sims's research shows that our "set point" works both ways, keeping our weight from going up as well as from going down.

The ecstasy of weight loss and agony of regain have been vividly portrayed by Gina Kolata in her book *Rethinking Thin*. She chronicled the weekly meetings of a group of obese men and women participating in a two-year weight-loss study and using either the Atkins or a low-fat diet. In the first session, each of the volunteers talked about their all-too-frequent experiences with losing and regaining weight and ending up heavier; still, all were optimistic that this time they would keep the lost pounds off. Over the next few months, all of them did lose weight, and they were buoyant and thrilled with their success. But then, as it almost always does, their weight loss stopped and they began to regain the weight they had lost, and their initial euphoria turned into anguish and dismay. In the end, the set point nearly always wins.

What Determines Our "Set Point" Weight?

Do you agree or disagree with this statement? "Some people are born to be fat and some thin; there is not much you can do to change this." If you are like most American women, you will disagree. When three thousand representative American women were recently asked this question, less than a third thought that this statement was true. Even two out of three overweight and obese women rejected the idea that our weights are largely inherited.

If a woman's weight is *not* mostly set when she is born, then she should be able to control how much she weighs. That would mean that thinner women must be those with the will and fortitude to do what is necessary to keep their weights down, while heavier women could be thin if they just tried harder. But this is simply not true. Our weights *are* pretty much set when we are born. We can see this by using the geneticist's favorite tool: comparing twins.

Separated at Birth

Jim Lewis and Jim Springer are identical twins separated when they were four weeks old and adopted by two different families far apart. Thirty-nine years later, they were reunited. Each had been married (twice) to women with the same first names, had a son with the same name, drove the same car, and held the same job. But in addition to all these curious similarities was a more interesting fact: After thirty-nine years apart, they both weighed exactly the same when they were reunited: 180 pounds. They weighed the same because they have the same genes and shared the same womb before they were born. The very different families that they grew up in had no effect on their weights.

Systematic studies of many pairs of identical twins reared apart in Denmark and in the United States show the same pattern; even though they grew up in different families, they tend to have very similar weights. This research suggests that more than two-thirds of the differences in weight between men and women are connected to the particular genes they have, while the homes where they are raised make little difference. So our genes together with our experience in our mother's womb account for most of our differences in weight. Our future set points are indeed largely determined by the time we are born.

We can also see this by looking at how women's weights at different times in their lives are related. When American women were asked in the early 1970s to give their lowest weight after turning eighteen, the average was 117 pounds. Half weighed between 105 and 125 pounds and more than two-thirds weighed between 100 and 130 pounds. This pattern of weights, with most clustered around the average, is what we expect to see when there are a number of different genes that influence weight.

But even though almost all of these young women were of "normal" weight in their late teens, how much they weighed in their teens still largely determined who would be normal weight, overweight, or obese when they reached their forties. Most of those whose low weight had been less than 110 still had normal weights a quarter of a century later; most who had weighed more than 125 became overweight; and most who had weighed more than 140 became obese. This shows that a woman's *relative* weight—whether she is heavier or lighter than others—stays pretty stable over her lifetime, because it is mostly controlled by her genes.

Now, with our recent dietary changes, the average weight has gone up, but the same rules about relative weights still apply. When American women were recently asked the same question about their low weight after eighteen, almost all had gained much more since age eighteen than the women polled in the 1970s. Nevertheless, how much they weighed now was still largely determined by their lowest weight in their late teens, just as it had been for women thirty years earlier.

So, much as we might wish it were otherwise, the natural "set point" for our weights is largely determined when we are born and there are severe limits to how much we can lower it. The very few women who maintain weights well below their set points are those who are willing to endure a perpetual state of semistarvation and a rigorous exercise regimen.

Dieting Causes Women to Gain Weight

Although our set points are largely determined at birth, there are unfortunately some things we can do to make our set points *increase*, and one of these is dieting to lose weight. Many studies have looked at the effect that dieting has on women's weights over time. They start by asking a group of women how often they have dieted in the past to lose weight and then they check back after a year or more to see how their weights have changed. All of these studies have found that the women who have dieted the most in the past gain more weight over time than the women who have dieted less. (It's hard to find women who have never dieted.) The more frequently women diet, the more they gain. For example, one of these studies followed a group of overweight nurses in their thirties for eight years. Almost all had dieted at some time in the previous four years, but those who had dieted more often and lost more weight during their diets gained ten pounds more over the eight years than those who had dieted less.

Why Dieting Raises the "Set Point" in Susan's Brain

The reason that women who use weight-loss diets tend to gain more weight than those who do not is that dieting sends a strong warning to the hypothalamus, telling it to store more fat for the future. Let's see how this works.

When Jeffrey was continuing to eat half as many calories a day as usual and losing less and less weight in Ancel Keys's laboratory, the part of his brain fighting to keep his weight from going down was the hypothalamus. As we saw in chapter 5, the hypothalamus is the part of the brain that controls a woman's appetite, determines the size of her children, and controls the set point for her weight, allowing her to gain weight after she's had a child.

Susan's typical almond-size hypothalamus is buried deep down in the bottom part of her brain and is one of its oldest and most primitive parts. In many animals, it is the main part of the brain. In its role as a sort of building supervisor for Susan's body, her hypothalamus is a full-time worrier. It is in charge of all of the most basic functions of her body, and it constantly checks up on everything to make sure it's all running right. It speeds up her heart when she is exercising and slows it down when she is resting. It cools her off when she is hot and warms her up when she is cold. If she's under stress, it tells her adrenal gland to make more stress hormone (cortisol). Acting through her pituitary gland, it controls her ovaries and thyroid gland and regulates her supply of growth hormone. It runs her sex life, too, telling her ovaries when to release an egg, her libido when to make love, her uterus when to start contracting, and her breasts when to make milk. It also keeps track of the time of day (and even the time of year), putting her to sleep at night and waking her up each morning.

As if that weren't enough of a job description for a nut-size bit of brain tissue, what Susan's hypothalamus worries most about is whether she has enough to eat and drink. This makes sense, because without food and water nothing else in her body works. It continually monitors the water level in her blood and makes her thirsty if it dips too low. To find out whether it's time for her to eat again, it constantly checks on how much leptin hormone is being released from her fat cells, how much insulin and sugar are in her blood, and how much food is in her stomach and intestine. When these signals agree that her supplies are low, it makes her feel hungry.

Susan's nervous hypothalamus considers sixty-eight pounds of fat to be the right amount for her; this is her "set point." When her fat cells have this much stored fat, they release twenty-two units of leptin into her blood. The level of her leptin is like a bank statement. It tells her brain what the current balance is in her fat account, and her brain works to keep her balance steady, just like a thermostat works to keep your home's temperature the same. When she is more active and burns more calories and her account balance goes down, her hypothalamus makes her hungrier until she pays back the deficit. If she eats more than usual or exercises less so that her fat and leptin increase, it makes her less hungry until the extra fat is used up.

Her brain also checks on how much daylight there is, so that it knows when there is likely to be more or less food available. And even though Susan has plenty to eat year-round, her hypothalamus always worries about whether she has enough food to meet the costs of having a baby. In countries where food is scarce during certain times of the year and more plentiful at others, like Bangladesh, women are much more likely to have their babies when food supplies are high. Even in today's America, women are more likely to give birth during the harvest season than in the dead of winter.

When she is eating normally, Susan stores most of her calories after a meal and releases some of them from storage in between her meals. About two-thirds of her calories normally come from the sugar and sugar compounds (starches) in her food. When the cells in her pancreas find that her blood sugar is going up, they pump out insulin hormone. As we saw in chapter 5, this insulin tells her cells to save sugar, fat, and amino acids. In between her meals, when her insulin goes back down, some of this stored sugar, fat, and amino acids is released back into her blood so that her cells can keep going until her next meal. And all of this storage and release are carefully regulated by her hypothalamus to help keep her weight in line with her set point.

So what happens when Susan goes on a weight-loss diet? Unfortunately, her hypothalamus has no way to know that she *wants* to lose weight. It's just the building supervisor; it's not on the board of directors, and it doesn't get memos about the board's high-level decisions. It just keeps doing its job of worrying, and it soon senses that less sugar is coming in and less insulin is being released from her pancreas. After a day or two, the sugar stored in her liver is used up and her insulin level falls even more. To make up for the missing calories, the drop in her insulin causes more of the fatty acids stored in her fat cells to be released back into her blood. Because this decreases her stored fat, her leptin level starts to drop. Meanwhile, the more of her fat that is used up, the happier Susan feels, because when she steps on the scale, she can see that her weight is going down; and when she puts on her slacks or jeans, she can feel that they are looser. The board of directors is quite pleased with this result.

But the building supervisor—her hypothalamus—isn't in the loop, and it's becoming increasingly concerned about her falling leptin levels. As long as Susan isn't losing too much weight too quickly, her hypothalamus is cautious about responding. It tells Susan she should be eating more, but it's not yet taking any drastic steps. During most of human history there have been times of year when food is plentiful, like summer, and times when supplies are low, like winter. In places where food supplies fluctuate and little food is stored, women may lose five to ten pounds during these lean months. So Susan's brain is willing to let some of her stored fat go without fighting too hard. In fact, if she starts her diet when the days are short (like New Year's Day), that's a time of the year when her hypothalamus expects that she might lose some weight.

If she is just having a limited seasonal weight loss, Susan's brain doesn't want to make it too difficult for her to work, to do what is necessary to make food available in the future. For example, in Bangladesh, there is less food available during the monsoon season and women like Yasmin often lose some weight; but there is still a lot of work to be done planting the next season's crops. So Susan feels hungry, but not too bad, and she is also quite happy to be losing weight.

But if she continues to lose weight or loses more than a pound a week, her hypothalamus begins to suspect that this may be a serious food shortage, a real famine, not just a normal seasonal fluctuation. The more weight she loses and the faster her pounds come off, the more suspicious and worried her hypothalamus becomes. What happens to Susan now is the same thing that happened to Jeffrey in Ancel Keys's laboratory, the obese dieters in Jules Hirsch's lab, and Gina Kolata's dieting group: Her brain hunkers down. Rather than just releasing more of her stored fat, her hypothalamus now takes several steps to reduce the number of calories she is using so that her weight loss will slow down. It uses fewer calories digesting her food. Her muscles work more efficiently than before. Through its control of her thyroid gland, her hypothalamus slows down her metabolism so that she is burning fewer calories to keep herself going. Her fat cells become more and more reluctant to let go of fat. Fewer of her calories are wasted as heat; every calorie becomes precious. At the same time, her brain also takes steps to make Susan less active. Just as it makes her feel sleepy at night, now it makes her feel tired and depressed all the time, and her activity level falls. But any time she thinks about food, her brain immediately gives her an emotional reward and so, like Jeffrey and the dieters in Hirsch's lab, she thinks about food more and more.

Because Susan is not really in the middle of a famine, these efforts of her hypothalamus will likely start to pay off. Her weight loss will slow down and then stop. Perhaps without her even realizing it, she will begin to eat more, with little snacks here and there; but her body is now in the mode of hoarding every calorie. Instead of losing weight, her weight will begin to creep up. And because she is no longer losing weight, she will no longer feel the delight she had when her fat was melting away; she will no longer have positive feelings to counterbalance the negative famine-fearing ones being generated by her hypothalamus. Deprivation is all that she'll feel. Because of all these actions by her hypothalamus, Susan will start to regain the weight she lost even though she may continue to try to limit her calories.

This is why Susan, and people in general, find it very difficult to keep weight off: Their hypothalamus is determined to get back at least to its normal leptin set point. But if Susan has managed to lose more than ten or fifteen pounds, she may not just regain the weight she lost. Because her hypothalamus is also concerned about her future needs, it will not be satisfied with going back to her old leptin level. It will want her to store more food against an uncertain future, and so it will *raise her set point*. Why? The lesson her hypothalamus has learned from Susan's diet is that her food supply is unreliable—that periods of severe shortage are likely to come again. As a direct response to this threat, it will push her to store more fat so that she will have a bigger cushion when famine strikes again. And every time she diets it will become more convinced that she lives in a world with an unreliable food supply. It does not matter what kind of diet Susan chooses; if it leads to significant weight loss then her hypothalamus will want her to be heavier. This is why dieters gain more weight than those who do not diet. The more often they diet and the more weight they lose, the more their brains want them to gain, to eat more when the eating is good.

This means that over the next several months, Susan is not only likely to regain the weight she lost, but to gain extra weight as well. She is likely to prefer foods with more calories. Studies show that the brain's reward centers light up for high-calorie foods after just sixteen hours of fasting. And like other women who diet frequently, Susan is likely to continue to have higher levels of the hormones that increase her appetite. Like them, she will also tend to store more of her calories as fat, burn less of it, and continue to have a slower metabolism. And her fat cells will continue to hold on to fat.

The more weight a woman loses with her diets, the higher her leptin set point will rise and the more weight she will be likely to gain to match this new set point. This increase in the leptin set point has been demonstrated in a study of a group of obese Italian women. The more cycles of weight loss and gain a woman had, the higher her leptin level was; the women who had lost the most weight before gaining it back had the highest leptin levels.

In addition to promoting even more weight gain, repeated dieting has other bad effects as well. Frequent dieting cycles—losing and regaining weight—may also increase blood pressure, decrease good cholesterol, increase inflammation, and even reduce life span. Dieting also tends to lead to more added waist fat more than fat in other areas. Women who diet frequently are also more likely to be depressed and have low self-esteem. Finally, during a diet, women may even have a decrease in mental ability. But if dieting doesn't work, what other options do you have?

What *Can* You Do to Have a Lower Weight?

Valerie Frankel tells a very instructive story about herself in her book *Thin Is the New Happy*. After many years of dieting, losing weight, and regaining more, she finally determined to get off the diet merry-go-round. She decided to stop dieting, weighing herself, and thinking about her weight all the time and just eat real foods when she was hungry and stop when she was full. Unexpectedly, she found that her weight *gradually* declined after she stopped dieting, and she went down two dress sizes in eleven months. Now that she was eating a healthy diet and not trying to lose weight by dieting—or regaining weight she had previously lost—her body spontaneously but slowly went down to her natural weight, the weight programmed for her when she was born. She is convinced that any woman can move down to her genetically programmed weight if she stops dieting, eats healthy foods, and changes her negative attitudes about eating and weight.

Graziella, a woman in the weight-loss study discussed by Gina Kolata, tells a similar story. Even as a child she was always quite heavy, just like the other women in her family, and dieted repeatedly without success. She started the study at 223 pounds and went down to 204 before she started gaining back the weight she had lost. She, too, finally decided to stop dieting, to choose natural and organic foods, and to eat only until she was satisfied: "I don't pick them because I have to. It's what I like eating now. It's become a part of me. This is not really a diet. It's a way of life." Using this approach she has stayed comfortably at 212 pounds. After a lifetime of dieting and increasing weight, she has now come to see that for her, this is a natural and healthy weight: "And why can't a woman be 212 pounds?"

Another woman's experience vividly shows how eating an unnatural American diet raises weight, while changing back to a more natural diet brings it back down. Nine years ago, Joanna moved to Pittsburgh from Katowice in southern Poland to study business and photography. She was twenty years old and weighed 115 pounds. In Katowice, she had typical home-cooked meals with soups, meats, lots of cabbage, bread, dairy, and potatoes, and these foods were often cooked with lots of animal fat.

Compared with our current American diet, the Polish diet has half as much vegetable oil, and most of that is canola oil, which is high in omega-3 and monounsaturated fat; there is very little soybean oil and no corn oil. Compared to Americans, the Poles eat three times more animal fats like butter and cream, two-thirds more cereal grains like wheat and rye, twice as many potatoes, a similar amount of meat but much more pork and much less chicken, about the same amount of vegetables, and a little less sugar. The average weight of adult women in Poland is 144 pounds, exactly the same as it was for American women in the early 1970s when our diet was more like that of Europeans.

After arriving in Pittsburgh, Joanna did some of her own cooking, and she shopped for meat, produce, and eggs in regular grocery stores, but she quickly noticed that they tasted much different from those back home and were much less appealing. Seeing "Polish ham" for sale in a deli, she eagerly bought some, only to find that it tasted more like plastic than the ham she had in Poland. Like most students, she also bought inexpensive prepared foods like donuts, pizza, and hot dogs.

When she first arrived here, her weight had been stable at 115 pounds for the previous three years and was typical of the young women in her school in Poland. None of them were obese and very few were overweight. In fact, no one she knew in Katowice was obese—much different from the people she saw in Pittsburgh. American visitors in Katowice were easy to tell from the Europeans, because the Americans were almost always heavier.

After just two months of eating American supermarket foods, Joanna's weight ballooned by twenty-four pounds; and when she went home for a visit, her mother was sure that she was ill because she looked so bloated. But after just a few weeks of eating her usual Polish diet— but *not* trying to lose weight—her extra weight disappeared. When she returned to Pittsburgh, she was determined to maintain a diet like the one she had in Poland and soon discovered that the meats and eggs sold here as "organic" tasted more like the everyday meat and eggs in Poland. So she decided to buy and prepare only organic foods and to avoid all processed and prepared foods (except for her favorite chocolate). With this approach, her weight stayed at 115 pounds until she gave birth to her daughter three years ago, after which she gained a few pounds as women usually do. Joanna's experience vividly illustrates the extent to which the typical American diet has diverged from the European diet over the past forty years and the dramatic effect of those changes on women's weights.

The alterations in the American diet over the past forty years combined with frequent dieting by many women have pushed our set points higher. Since dieting doesn't work, the most important step we can take to return to our naturally lower weights is to stop dieting and take steps to reverse the changes in our diet that have led us to consume too much omega-6 fat and too little omega-3.

Earlier we saw that a woman stores large amounts of lower-body fat during childhood and youth to provide omega-3 DHA for her children's brains and that her set point tends to rise after she has her first child so that she will gain more weight and benefit her younger children. But the unnatural changes in our diet and frequent dieting have pushed our set points much higher than is usual. Where Susan's set point would have been sixteen units of leptin in the past, it is now twenty-two.

As we have seen, one reason for this change is that the increase in omega-6 fat and decrease in omega-3 fat in the American diet makes it much harder for women to store the amount of omega-3 DHA they need for their children's brains. Since the proportion of DHA in their stored fat is lower, they need to store more fat to have the same total amount of DHA available. The very low levels of omega-3 in our blood may be constantly telling our brains that we need to store more fat, thus pushing our set points higher.

Another result of our severe imbalance of omega-6 and omega-3 fat is that we make more of the signaling molecules (eicosanoids) and marijuana-like endocannabinoids that come from omega-6 arachidonic. A chronic increase in these levels in our blood, combined with low levels of omega-3, may also cause our hypothalamus to raise our set points; and this has been shown in animals. Both of these possibilities arise from the same cause: too much omega-6 and too little omega-3 in our diets. And to the degree that this is responsible for increasing our set points, it should be possible to counteract this effect by restoring a proper balance through decreasing the omega-6 and increasing the omega-3 that we eat, just as Joanna went back to her usual weight when she returned to a more natural diet.

By returning to a diet more like that of Americans in the past and Europeans today, much of our extra weight should come off. Your weight may not be as low as you would like it to be, but you should be closer to your natural weight. The best way to achieve this weight loss is by making a permanent change to a better overall diet rather than by dieting to lose weight. If you are eating the right foods and getting a reasonable amount of exercise, your weight should find its natural level. We will show you how to achieve your natural set-point weight in the rest of this book. We'll provide specific suggestions on how to choose foods so that you can avoid omega-6 and increase omega-3, as well as other ways to bring your set point more in line with your natural weight. We will also suggest ways to estimate what your natural weight and shape are likely to be if you follow this plan.

The very first step in starting a new approach to your body is to accept that dieting doesn't work, just as Valerie and Graziella did. Dieting has not worked in the past, and it's not likely that any new approach to dieting is going to work any better. All of the recent diet crazes, including the Atkins and South Beach diets, were first tried more than a hundred years ago, and they didn't work then either. It is possible that a drug company will come up with a weight-loss drug that is safe, effective, and free of serious side effects. They are certainly doing their best to find one. But what we know about the brain suggests that the control of our appetites by the hypothalamus is too complex and has too many backup systems to be tricked by any simple drug. If one part of the appetite system is blocked, another part is likely to work harder to compensate. Only changing the set point is likely to be effective, and since our unnatural diet and our dieting have raised our set points, only permanently returning to a more natural diet will allow them to fall and reverse our excessive weight gains. In the next two chapters we will look at what changes you need to make to accomplish this, and then we will show you how to determine what your natural weight and shape are likely to be if you make these changes.

CHAPTER 8

What to Eat

As we saw in chapter 2, over the past forty years Americans have been eating much more high-omega-6 vegetable oils than in the past while consuming unusually low amounts of omega-3 fat. That dietary change—more than any other—has led to our expanding waistlines. Not only does omega-6 cause increased weight gain, but it greatly interferes with our ability to extract and use the little omega-3 there is in our diet. That's especially bad because these omega-3s are critical; they help to *decrease* our weights and are essential to our brain performance and health. In the diet of our Stone Age ancestors there was probably more omega-3 than omega-6; in the current American diet, we have more than *twenty times* as much omega-6 as omega-3. Having more bad fat *and* less good fat in our diet is the perfect storm for weight gain.

The best way to undo this damage and help your body find its natural weight is to reduce the amount of omega-6 in the foods that you eat and, at the same time, increase omega-3 foods. A large part of the excess omega-6 in our diets—as much as four-fifths—comes from foods prepared by others, including meals eaten away from home and processed or prepared convenience foods. Collectively, our weights have climbed as these foods have increasingly dominated our diets. The best way to ensure that your diet is on the right track is to eat real, unprocessed foods and prepare them in a way that minimizes omega-6 and maximizes omega-3.

Pushing Down Omega-6

One helpful step in reducing omega-6 is to reduce the commercially fried foods in your diet. Most are fried in either corn or soybean oil, both of which are very high in omega-6 and might still contain some trans fats, and these oils add up to thirty-two pounds of cooking oil for each American per year. Omega-6 is apt to be high in most ready-to-eat fried foods like potato or tortilla chips as well as restaurant or fast foods that are fried, like french fries, onion rings, chicken, and fish. Because of their high omega-6 and low omega-3 content, corn and soybean oil are two of the *worst* possible frying fats; but they are used by the food industry because they are cheap, stable, and can be used over and over. Some foods, like potatoes, absorb a lot of this fat when they are cooked. Others that soak up less oil on their own—like meats, poultry, or fish—are often covered in breading or batter before they are fried, which greatly increases the amount of oil they absorb in the cooking process.

For these reasons, one simple way to cut down on omega-6 is to reduce the amount of commercial fried foods that you eat. Instead you can cook without fat by boiling, roasting, steaming, stewing, broiling, or grilling or look for foods prepared in this way. If you crave the taste of something fried, try sautéing, stir-frying, or braising in a low-omega-6 oil such as canola or olive oil or in butter; it will give you a similar (or better) taste without a big dose of omega-6. How food is prepared is critical not only because it can contribute a lot of extra omega-6, but also because of the competition between omega-6 and omega-3 fats. For example, even though fish is usually an excellent source of omega-3, if it is breaded and fried in corn or soybean oil, its good fats are overwhelmed and blocked by the big dose of omega-6 fats from the frying process.

Although most processed and prepared food products are also made with soybean or corn oil, oils that are very high in omega-6, it is often difficult to know this for certain because of a loophole in the labeling law. Instead of telling you what oils their foods actually contain, food labels often say that they "may contain" two or more different oils. For example, the phrase "may contain soybean or canola oil" is quite common. Manufacturers say that they do this so that they can use whatever oil is available at the best price at the time they make the product. But, because of this labeling loophole, there is no way to know which oil will be in the product you buy. This labeling practice is harmfully deceptive; manufacturers know that some consumers will want a product with canola oil or olive oil, and the law unfortunately lets them gratuitously list it on the label without ever putting it in their product!

If a label says that it "may contain" harmful high-omega-6/low-omega-3 oils, like soybean and corn oil, it almost certainly does, while it is much less likely to have regular canola oil, which is high in omega-3. Processed-food makers prefer high-omega-6/low-omega-3 oils because they are cheaper and much less perishable. Omega-6 has a much longer shelf life than omega-3. So they are unlikely to be putting a lot of high-omega-3 oil, like regular canola, in any product that sits on grocery shelves. Products enriched in omega-3 like certain eggs or margarines need to be refrigerated. To make matters worse, there are now low-omega-3 types of "high-stability" canola oils, so even if a product says that it contains canola oil, it may not be the good kind. Canola oil may also be hydrogenated when used in processed foods. It is best to avoid products which "may contain" more than one oil and to limit processed foods with added oils as much as possible.

Reducing all forms of omega-6 fat in our diets is critical if we are to return to our natural weights. As we have seen, omega-6 fat comes in two forms in foods. The kind in vegetable oil is *linoleic*. In our bodies, we convert this linoleic to *arachidonic*, the form that actually causes weight gain, promotes inflammation, and is generally unhealthy. The major sources of omega-6 *linoleic* in our current diet are meats, chicken, and fish that are fried or served with other oily foods (30 percent of dietary linoleic), baked goods (23 percent), salad dressings and margarines (16 percent), and french fries and potato chips (8 percent). Some foods also contain preformed *arachidonic*, and the major sources of this in the American diet include poultry (45 percent of dietary arachidonic), red meats (25 percent), and regular eggs (12 percent). To minimize excessive weight gain, you should try to reduce the amount of both types of omega-6 in your diet as much as possible.

Pushing Up Omega-3

On the other side of the equation is omega-3 fat, the good fat that opposes weight gain and promotes good brain function and health—the fat that we need more of. As we have seen, the most basic form of omega-3 is *alpha-linolenic*, which we can convert in our bodies into EPA and DHA, though not very well. EPA and DHA are the forms of omega-3 that our brain and body require and that make us healthier in other ways, such as reducing heart disease and inflammation, and getting them directly from our diet is the best way to make sure we get enough.

How much omega-3 should we have? Expert groups of scientists from around the world have recommended that all adults should have at least 250 milligrams a day of DHA and the same amount of EPA. However, higher levels may be even more beneficial, and some experts recommend more than four times as much for those with an American diet. The Japanese, who enjoy the highest life expectancy in the world and have very low rates of heart disease and obesity, average more than a gram (1,000 milligrams) of DHA and a bit less EPA in their daily diet, and a gram a day has also been shown to be safe in clinical studies. In fact, DHA is likely to be safe in amounts up to three times as high (3,000 milligrams a day), although you should talk to your physician before taking very large amounts.

While the recommended *minimum* amount of DHA is 250 milligrams a day, the government estimates that there are only 90 milligrams a day of DHA per person in the American food supply. The food histories of adult American women show that they average even less—only 70 milligrams a day. This level is very low: much less than one-third of the recommended minimum amount, and less than one-fourteenth of what the Japanese—whose children lead the world in math and science—are eating.

To make matters worse, much of the EPA and DHA in the American diet comes from corn-fed chickens and their eggs; and corn-based feeds result in much more of the competing omega-6 arachidonic in their meat than EPA and DHA. And the small amount of omega-3 they contain may not even be available to us when these foods are cooked with vegetable oils, as happens when fish is cooked with high-omega-6 oils. Because there is so much omega-6 in the American diet and stored away in our body fat, the optimal daily amount of DHA for American women is probably closer to 1,000 milligrams, plus a similar amount of EPA.

In addition to increasing EPA and DHA in our diets, it is also desirable to increase alpha-linolenic, the simplest form of omega-3. Just as we make omega-6 arachidonic from linoleic, we can also make omega-3 EPA and DHA out of alpha-linolenic, although the conversion process is very inefficient and is blocked by large amounts of omega-6. Major sources in our diet include canola oil, dairy foods, vegetables, fruits, and meats. Flax seeds and flax seed oil are the best sources.

By decreasing omega-6 and increasing omega-3 in our diets, we should be able to move back toward the natural weights that our genes intended for us. With this in mind, let's look more closely at each of the major food groups to see which specific foods are high in omega-6 and should be avoided and what foods are high in omega-3 and can help us to both improve our health and maintain a lower weight.

Meat and Dairy

Beef, Pork, Lamb, Chicken, and Eggs

By themselves, red meats are around 1 percent omega-6 linoleic, while chicken with the skin is roughly 3 percent. But meats are also the main source of omega-6 arachidonic in our diet, which may be one reason why higher meat consumption is linked to heavier weights. Women in countries with more beef, lamb, and poultry in the national diet tend to be heavier. Poultry meats (especially chicken) have the highest amounts of arachidonic and are the most strongly linked to higher weights. Heavier American women eat more beef, pork, lamb, chicken, and turkey than their lighter counterparts, and more meat overall. American women with higher levels of arachidonic in their diet are very likely to be heavier. Other studies also show higher weights in women who eat larger amounts of meat and have larger amounts of arachidonic in their diets. Vegetarians tend to weigh less than meat-eaters.

Unfortunately, the meats that most Americans eat today are quite different from those that we had in the past or than those in Europe (as Joanna from Poland discovered). Most of the animals we use for food evolved to eat grass. Like most green plants, grass is rich in omega-3 and has seven times more omega-3 than omega-6. The first grasslands appeared about 50 million years ago, and the ancestors of many of our modern farm animals took advantage of this new source of food. Until recently these farm animals were put out to pasture to eat grass, just like their wild ancestors, and grass was also cut, dried, and stored to feed them in the winter in the form of hay.

Unfortunately, since government subsidies created an abundance of cheap corn and soybeans in the 1950s, these have largely taken the place of grass for feeding livestock. Corn, a seed, has thirty-three times more omega-6 than omega-3. Feeding animals corn rather than grass not only increases the amount of both forms of omega-6—arachidonic and linoleic—in their meat, it also decreases the amount of beneficial omega-3 they contain. Corn-fed supermarket beef has seven times more omega-6 than omega-3, while in grass-fed beef omega-6 and omega-3 are almost equal.

As Michael Pollan has said, "You are what you eat eats." Both the good and bad elements of our animal feeding practices land on our plates. Our farm animals inevitably incorporate whatever we feed them into their flesh, milk, and eggs. Animals fed high-omega-6 diets will give that omega-6 right back to us in concentrated form. The stockyard-reared, corn-fed meats that dominate American supermarkets have no EPA or DHA, just arachidonic. In contrast, wild game animals, like elk and deer, have substantial amounts of EPA and DHA in their meat and much less arachidonic. Wild animals are, after all, the animals our Stone Age ancestors ate. Grass-fed cattle and bison also have DHA and EPA in their meat. But because our farm animals today are fed so much corn, their meats are much higher in omega-6 arachidonic while EPA and DHA are absent.

Choosing meats from grass-fed and free-range animals can help to improve your omega fat balance, and grass-fed beef has been found to be less likely to cause weight gain. It is probably best to eat typical supermarket meats from corn-fed animals only in moderation, to choose lean cuts, and to trim off visible fat. Remember, this is not because fat is bad. It's because rearing animals in the now-standard feedlot way causes them to store a heavy dose of omega-6 in their fat from the corn they are eating.

Regular supermarket chicken and turkey have even more omega-6 and a higher proportion of arachidonic than any other meat, and they account for almost half of the excessive arachidonic in our diets. Chickens and turkeys also naturally have significant amounts of DHA and EPA in their muscles, because these omega-3 fats help the muscles of birds to work better. Unfortunately, because they are now also fed mostly corn, there is fifteen times more omega-6 in their meat than omega-3. Poultry were supposed to be healthier than other meats because they have more polyunsaturated fat, and we now eat two and a half times more than we did forty years ago. However, heavier American women eat even more poultry than lighter women, especially chicken, and women's weights are higher in countries where more poultry is eaten.

Chickens that eat grass outdoors have twice as much omega-3 in their meat as grain-fed chickens and a ratio of omega-3 to omega-6 that is twice as high; pasture-fed chickens also have much higher levels of beneficial omega-3 EPA and DHA. So they are preferable even though they cost more. As with other meats, regular supermarket poultry is best eaten in moderation, without the skin, and with as much fat as possible removed before cooking.

Chicken eggs are also naturally high in DHA and EPA, but the high-omega-6 feeds that most chickens are now given also greatly decrease the amount of omega-3 while increasing the amount of omega-6 arachidonic. As a result, eggs are the source of one-eighth of the arachidonic in our diets. Chickens given feeds higher in omega-3, like grass, flaxseeds, or fish oil, produce eggs with much more omega-3 and much less omega-6, and these high-omega-3 eggs are also preferable despite their higher cost. Eggs from chickens fed flaxseeds each have around 100 milligrams of DHA, and those from chickens fed fish oil can have much more. Omega-3-enriched eggs also have substantially less omega-6 arachidonic and a much lower ratio of omega-6 to omega-3. Unfortunately, the producers of omega-3-enriched eggs do not always reveal their DHA content. If they give only the total amount of omega-3, you can assume that about one-fifth is DHA.

To make matters worse, when meat, poultry, and eggs are prepared in restaurants or as part of packaged foods, even more vegetable fat is usually added and the amount of omega-6 doubles or triples! Meats in combination with breads, starches, pasta, and other "helpers" account for a fifth of the omega-6 linoleic in the American diet. This includes meat in sandwiches, pizzas, quesadillas, burritos, and tacos from fast food vendors or made with prepackaged mixes. Although some people think that chicken sandwiches are healthier than hamburgers, fast-food chicken sandwiches contribute the most omega-6 linoleic in the sandwich group. Deli meats, breakfast meats, and sausages are also high in omega-6 linoleic. These high-linoleic foods are all eaten more often by heavier women.

Like other fried foods, fried chicken is quite high in omega-6, as is chicken with coatings (including fast-food chicken). Surprisingly, chicken cooked at home with packaged coatings can be even higher in omega-6. Precooked chicken, such as rotisserie chicken, is often injected with vegetable fat, as are some raw chicken and turkey parts sold in supermarkets; always check the label for any additives or "enrichments." Fast-food eggs served with biscuits or muffins for breakfast are also very high in linoleic, as are egg salad and deviled eggs.

Other prepared meat dishes high in linoleic include chicken or turkey pot pie, chicken or beef with noodles, dumplings, and many spaghetti sauces with meat. Many popular prepared Asian dishes are also high in linoleic, although those made with cornstarch, like beef with broccoli, are better than meats that are battered. Most commercially made Mexican meat dishes are also high in linoleic. Weight-conscious women often opt for salads, but unfortunately, prepared salads with tuna, chicken, or turkey are also high in linoleic because they are made with dressings very high in omega-6. Making your own salad from a salad bar is better if you choose a dressing low in omega-6, such as those made with olive oil.

Fish and Seafood

Fish and seafood ought to be the perfect foods. Unlike other types of animal foods, they have an ideal fat content. They are naturally low in omega-6 and have very large amounts of omega-3 DHA and EPA, because the algae at the base of the aquatic food chain can make these omega-3 fats from scratch and provide them to all animals that live in water. The high levels of DHA that fish get from these algae allow them to be active in cold water even though they are cold-blooded. The levels of DHA and EPA in different fish and seafoods are given in our "Fish and Seafood" table on pages 207–9. Women who eat more *nonfried* fish tend to weigh less, as do women in countries with more fish in the diet. Unfortunately—and this is very important—when fish is fried or coated in batter or cooked with other foods containing vegetable oil, the beneficial omega-3 that the fish contains is no longer available.

Since fish that is breaded or coated (like fish sticks) or fried does not provide omega-3, eating fish that is cooked with vegetable oils is linked with *higher* rather than lower weights. Heavier women tend to eat less fish overall, and the fish they do eat (mostly fast food) has *three times* as much omega-6 because of the way it is prepared. So heavier women not only eat less of the foods with the most DHA but are much less likely to get whatever DHA is in those foods. The best way to maximize DHA and EPA from fish and seafood (as with other meats) is to have it prepared without any added vegetable fat, by boiling, baking, broiling, steaming, stewing, or grilling. When fish and seafood are prepared in these ways, they are strongly linked with lower weights.

Unfortunately, *all* fish and seafood, perhaps the most beneficial foods that we can eat, are contaminated with mercury, a potent poison that can damage the brain and nerves. The same algae that make EPA and DHA also have the unfortunate ability to collect and concentrate any mercury present in the water, especially methyl mercury, the most toxic form. Most of the mercury in rivers, lakes, and oceans comes from the discharges of coal-burning power plants into the air that eventually come back down in rain, so water everywhere is affected—one of many good reasons to burn less coal. Thus, all fish and seafood have some mercury, and the amounts found in different types are given in our "Fish and Seafood" table on pages 207–9. Shark, swordfish, king mackerel, and tilefish have very high mercury levels and should be avoided. Salmon, trout, light tuna, pollock, sardines, herring, and perch are fish which are *relatively* low in mercury and high in omega-3 and so are good choices. However, to avoid their getting excessive amounts of mercury, the U.S. Food and Drug Administration recommends that women in their childbearing years should eat no more than twelve ounces of even "low-mercury" fish per week.

Another question about fish is whether it's wild-caught or farmed. While both types of salmon and trout have similar amounts of DHA, the DHA in farmed fish actually comes from fish oil from ocean fish that is added to their food. Fish cannot live without lots of DHA in their diet, normally from algae. Currently, more than half of all the fish oil harvested from the sea is fed to farmed fish. So taking fish-oil capsules instead of eating farmed fish would seem to be a much more efficient and environmentally sound choice. Farmed fish may also have high levels of other pollutants, like PCBs. Also, because of the other foods that farmed fish are fed, such as vegetable oils, they are likely to have more omega-6 than wild-caught fish, especially farmed tilapia and catfish. As a result, eating these may interfere with our absorption of the DHA they contain and add to our heavy omega-6 burden.

Fish Oils

While increasing omega-3 DHA and EPA in our diets is very important, getting enough from fish and seafood while avoiding mercury can be difficult. Because mercury is such a potent nervous system poison, even the "low" levels of mercury in preferred fish and seafood might still cause subtle, long-term health problems, which limits the amount of these foods that can be eaten. In addition, our bodies also store mercury in our fat. These risks are also likely to be even greater during pregnancy and nursing, because a developing baby is more vulnerable than an adult.

Women who wish to avoid such risks for themselves and their families should consider using fish oils in capsule or liquid form as a source of omega-3 EPA and DHA. These supplements are a much better source of omega-3s than secondhand fish oil from farmed fish. Reputable suppliers of fish oil and fish-oil capsules purify their product to eliminate mercury and other pollutants. Although the major brands of fish oil are purified in this way, it is best to check the bottle to make sure and, if in doubt, to contact the manufacturer. Some women find that taking fish oil before a meal reduces the amount of food they need to eat to feel satisfied, supporting the idea that American women now crave fat because they are not getting enough omega-3.

The total number of milligrams of *oil* in a fish-oil capsule, such as 1,000 or 1,200, is not very informative. The crucial question is how much DHA and EPA each capsule contains, and the label usually gives this information, though sometimes it (annoyingly) lumps them together. Also be sure to check how many capsules are in the serving size to see just how much omega-3 is in each one. Regular fish-oil capsules usually each have around 120 milligrams of DHA and a similar amount of EPA, while "double-strength" or "one-a-day" capsules have twice as much; "triple-strength" capsules are also available. Krill oil supplements also provide DHA and EPA but tend to have less DHA, cost more, and may not be purified. As we said earlier, the optimal daily amount of DHA for most American women is probably at least 500 to 1,000 milligrams.

If the size of fish oil capsules is a problem, you can chew them or puncture the capsule and squeeze out the oil onto a spoon. The oil is actually quite mild in flavor, and chewing the capsules releases the oil and reduces their size. The gelatin part melts away in a short time or can be easily swallowed. If you find that regular fish oil capsules increase burping, you can take the enteric-coated type, but these are less appealing to chew. Capsules can also be swallowed more easily if they are taken with a large portion of water. Another option is to buy fish oil in liquid form. Because DHA and EPA react so readily with the oxygen in the air, liquid oils must be kept in a dark bottle, refrigerated, and opened as little as possible.

Cod liver oil, which mothers often wisely gave to their children in bygone days, is an excellent source of DHA and EPA as well as vitamin D, but it also has quite a bit of vitamin A. Two teaspoons of cod liver oil have 1,000 milligrams of DHA but also 2,700 micrograms of vitamin A, which is close to the recommended daily *maximum* of vitamin A for women, so it is probably best not to have more than this each day. Studies in Norwegian women have found reduced cancer rates in those who take cod liver oil, and, as we would expect, they are also less likely to be obese. For strict vegetarians, DHA from algae is also available. This eliminates the "middleman" (fish), since all of the DHA in fish or seafood is made by algae. However, the EPA content of algae-based supplements may be lower.

Some omega-3 supplements combine DHA and EPA with alpha-linolenic, and these are acceptable as long as they contain adequate amounts of DHA and EPA, which are the active forms that we need the most. Supplements that contain just alpha-linolenic, such as those made with flaxseed oil, may also be beneficial in boosting omega-3, but they should not be substituted for those with DHA and EPA because the conversion of alpha-linolenic to DHA is very inefficient. A daily intake of one to two grams of alpha-linolenic is desirable.

Dairy Foods and Vitamin D

Because of the misguided dietary recommendations of the 1970s, Americans have cut down on most kinds of dairy foods. Whole milk, cream, and butter are feared because of their high saturated fat content, though we seem to be less afraid of cheese, which is also high in saturates. Europeans—particularly the notoriously healthy French—consume much more dairy than we do, especially butter, cream, and natural cheese (made directly from milk). Lighter American women also consume more dairy foods overall, drink more milk, and eat more yogurt and natural cheese than heavier women. Heavier women use more cream substitutes (often higher in omega-6) and eat more ice cream. Studies support the idea that dairy foods may help to reduce women's weights. Contradicting the saturated-fat myth, dairy foods are also linked to better general health. And because milk is rich in calcium, higher intakes of milk and dairy foods are also linked to lower risks of broken bones in the spine and hip. Milk and dairy foods also have a very good balance between omega-6 and omega-3 fats and contain no arachidonic. Milk from grass-fed animals is even better. Dairy foods also contain small amounts of natural trans fats, but unlike those that come from hydrogenated oils, these may be beneficial.

But what about the saturated fat in dairy foods? Countries with more saturated fat in their food supply today tend to have *lower* death rates from coronary disease, though their diets differ in many other ways as well. European countries have lower death rates from coronary heart disease than the United States and most have *higher* levels of saturated fat in their diets. France has the fourth-lowest coronary disease rate in the world and the French eat one-fifth *more* saturated fat per person than we do. A recent extensive review of all the studies of the relationship between dietary saturated fat and heart disease found no evidence that saturated fat increases coronary disease. Nor is saturated fat intake connected to cholesterol in the blood in women. Almost half the fat in a mother's milk is saturated, and there is a higher percentage than in cow's milk. Having sufficient omega-3 in the diet is much more beneficial to health—and heart health in particular—than any decrease in saturated fat.

Most dairy products are also enriched with vitamin D, and this vitamin is also linked to lower weights: The more vitamin D American women have in their blood, the less they tend to weigh, and the amount of milk a woman drinks is strongly related to her blood levels of this vitamin. Vitamin D deficiency seems to be a growing problem in the United States, with blood levels lower now than they were in 1990. So increasing dairy products in your diet may also help to lower your weight by increasing vitamin D. Of course, you can also make your own vitamin D by exposing some of your skin to sunlight for a few minutes a day. Fish also have moderate amounts of vitamin D, and cod liver oil is an excellent source of both vitamin D and omega-3.

Vegetables, Grains, and Fruits

Vegetables and fruits are the original source of omega-3 for animals that live on land. The process by which plants convert sunlight into energy (photosynthesis) requires omega-3 alpha-linolenic in the plant cell membrane and comparatively little omega-6 linoleic. So most green plants have more omega-3 than omega-6 fat, though the amounts are quite small. In their natural state—without extensive processing—fruits and vegetables have generally less than 1 percent fat, with about a tenth of a percent of omega-3 alpha-linolenic; we would have to eat a very large amount to get all the omega-3 we need. Since vegetables and fruits have a good balance between omega-3 and omega-6 even though the amounts are relatively small, having more of them in our diets is beneficial.

Fruits, vegetables, and grains are also the main source of fiber in our diets, mostly in the form of carbohydrates that we cannot digest. Women with diets higher in vegetable fiber tend to have lower weights. About half of our fiber comes from grains, a third from other vegetables, a sixth from fruit, and a bit less from nuts. Although the recommended amount is twenty to thirty-five grams a day, American women average only fourteen grams of fiber a day. Only one woman in seven eats twenty grams or more, but those who do tend to weigh less. Several other studies also show that heavier women have lower fiber intake, typically five to ten grams less than lighter women. And fiber is not only beneficial for weight, it seems to be good for overall health. Several studies show that women with higher fiber intakes tend to live longer than those with lower intakes. Fiber supplements may also help to lower women's weights.

Potatoes: A Surprising Source of Omega-6

Roots like potatoes have been a major source of calories in human diets for many thousands of years. Plain potatoes by themselves are less than 1 percent omega-6 and, like most vegetables, have some omega-3, and so are a good diet choice. Yet potatoes account for 8 percent of our linoleic intake. How can that be? It's because we now eat most of our potatoes in the form of chips and french fries soaked with vegetable fat. A single potato chip or french fry has almost a half gram of omega-6, so it adds up quickly. Baked chips generally have less fat than regular fried potato chips. Making your own fries or chips with canola or olive oil or baking them without fat is preferable. A few brands of chips fried in olive oil are also now available. Always beware of the "may contain one of the following oils" trap; if there are any high-omega-6 oils on the list, like soybean or corn oil, that's almost certainly the one that was used, because these oils are cheaper and less perishable.

Not long ago, Lay's potato chips had an advertising campaign built around the phrase "Bet you can't eat just one!" If you eat a medium-size baked potato with butter or sour cream, it is generally satisfying. You don't usually feel as if you must have another right away. But when you eat potato chips or french fries, they do not seem to satisfy us in the same way. Even though each chip or french fry has an abundance of fat and almost a half gram of linoleic, we tend to keep eating them; they are appealing but not satisfying. Potato chips made with lard are more filling. So it seems that omega-6 vegetable fats do not satisfy us in the same way as the animal fats that were our major sources of dietary fat during our Stone Age past, and this leads us to eat more and contributes to our gaining weight.

Other Fruits and Vegetables

While many diets encourage eating lots of vegetables to help lose weight, the total amount of vegetables in a woman's diet is generally not strongly related to women's weights in different countries, in American women, or in most diet-and-weight studies. Lighter women do tend to have more fruit, a greater variety of fruits, and much more dried fruit and berries. Having more fruit in the diet has also been linked with lower weights in other studies. Higher amounts of vitamin C in American women's blood are strongly linked with lower weights, and all citrus fruits, like oranges, lemons, and limes, are high in vitamin C, with smaller amounts in other fruits and vegetables.

In addition to vitamin C, we also find that certain other nutrients in American women's blood that come from certain fruits and vegetables are strongly related to lower weights, and some other studies have also found this. These are the colored nutrients: orange carotenes and yellow xanthins. Carotenes and xanthins can be transformed into vitamin A, a fat-soluble vitamin that supports vision and cell growth, and these colored nutrients are also "antioxidants" that help to get rid of damaging forms of oxygen in our cells. The diet records of American women who weigh less show higher intakes of these nutrients, and lighter women also eat more yellow, dark green, and raw vegetables, such as leaf lettuce, carrots, squash, and tomatoes, as well as more of many kinds of fruit. When measured in women's blood, the relationship of these nutrients to lower weights is much stronger, probably because blood values more accurately reflect what people actually eat than their diet records do.

Although these nutrients are found in most fruits and vegetables, as a rule of thumb, those that are strongly colored, such as those that are dark green, orange, red, yellow, or purple, are the richest sources. These include carrots, greens, chard, kale, leaf lettuce, peppers, olives, and spinach as well as fruits like mango, apricots, cantaloupe, papaya, persimmons, and tangerines.

Some forms of these nutrients, such as beta-carotene and vitamin C, may be included in certain vitamin supplements. But most of the nutrients in our blood that are strongly linked to lower weights are not found in supplements and so must be coming from the fruits and vegetables in our diets. In addition, supplements do not seem to have the same benefits as the natural antioxidants in food. For example, while fruits and vegetables high in beta-carotene reduce the risk of cancer, beta-carotene supplements do not.

Unfortunately, when vegetables are eaten with high-omega-6 vegetable oils their weight-lowering value may be lost, just as these oils block the omega-3 in fish. Women who have high blood levels of gamma-tocopherol, indicating a higher intake of soybean and corn oil, have lowered blood levels of the beneficial vitamins. Heavier American women are much more likely to eat vegetables in dishes prepared with high-omega-6 oils, and this probably interferes with their ability to absorb the valuable nutrients they contain.

In addition to the nutrients in vegetables, the fiber they contain may also help to lower our weights. Beans are especially rich in fiber; kidney, black, lima, navy, and great northern beans have six or seven grams per serving. Peas, lentils, Brussels sprouts, and potatoes with the skin are also high in fiber. Carrots, broccoli, cauliflower, peppers, eggplant, potatoes, and spinach are moderately high, while tomatoes have a bit less. Beginning a meal with a salad or other food high in fiber, like a vegetable dish, may reduce the number of calories eaten in a meal.

Most fruits are moderately high in fiber, and fruit supplies about one-sixth of the fiber in the diets of American women. Fruits with larger amounts include apples, bananas, oranges, grapefruit, pears, prunes, blackberries, and raspberries, while melons, nectarines, peaches, and plums have a little less. Since fruits and vegetables are rich in fiber and other beneficial nutrients, including the antioxidant carotenes and vitamin C, as well as having a high ratio of omega-3 to omega-6, they are desirable for many reasons.

Since so many of the foods we like are supposed to be bad for us, it is a pleasant surprise to discover that chocolate from cocoa beans—long regarded with horror by nutritionists—may actually have some health benefits and may help to reduce weight. However, it's important to realize that this applies only to dark chocolate, not to milk chocolate. Milk can interfere with the absorption of flavonoids, the specific ingredients in chocolate (and wine) that seem to provide their unique health benefits. Although Americans have been eating more chocolate than we used to, we still lag well behind the slimmer French, who eat about a third more. Chocolate may be especially useful at the end of a meal by increasing our feeling of being satisfied. The dark chocolate mousse made with omega-3-enriched eggs pictured on the cover is an excellent choice, providing almost as much DHA as a typical fish-oil capsule in a delectable form. There is also some evidence that chocolate may decrease the risk of heart disease, high blood pressure, inflammation, and cancer.

Baked Goods, Grains, Cereals, Rice, and Pasta

Flour made from wheat has much less than 1 percent omega-6 linoleic along with a very small amount of omega-3, yet a quarter of all the linoleic in our diets comes from baked goods. The reason these contribute so much is that most baked goods contain shortening made from soybean oil, and these shortenings add up to twenty-two pounds for each American per year. Because of this vegetable shortening, commercial baked goods are usually high in omega-6 linoleic and contain little omega-3 alpha-linolenic. Also, until recently, commercial baked goods usually also contained a lot of trans fat, and many of those made with shortening probably still have some. Food makers can say "zero" trans fat on the label if a "serving" contains less than one-half gram. A label for cookies that each contain a half gram of trans fat can state "zero trans fat" as long as the serving size listed is one cookie.

Breads account for almost half of the linoleic from baked goods. White bread is fairly high in linoleic, and sweet rolls, biscuits, muffins, and bread sticks are higher; all are eaten more frequently by heavier women. Commercial cakes, cookies, pastries, and pies are also high in linoleic, and heavier women eat more cake. Breads and baked goods made with whole wheat, rye, or oats tend to be a little lower in omega-6 (and higher in fiber) and are more popular with lighter women. Bagels, sourdough, rye, and pita breads also tend to have less omega-6 and French and sprouted-grain breads have little or no oil; check the label. You can also ask at bakeries about the oils they use. Delicious home-made breads can be made with canola and olive oils; automatic bread-making machines work well and greatly simplify the process of home baking. Salty snacks, such as corn puffs, crackers, and corn popped in oil, are quite high in linoleic and heavier women tend to eat more of these foods as well.

Like plain potatoes and wheat, rice and pasta are low in omega-6 linoleic and can be eaten without any restrictions. Brown rice and regular pasta are also moderately high in fiber, and pastas made with whole grains are even better. Breakfast cereals made with wheat or oats generally have 1 to 2 percent omega-6, though oatmeal has less.

Sugars and Sweeteners

Sugars are fat free and have fifteen calories per teaspoon. As we saw earlier, the share of calories from sugar has actually decreased in the American diet. However, if we look at different countries, women do tend to weigh more when there is more sugar in the national diet. We have a bigger calorie share from sugar than France, but about the same share as Denmark, Belgium, and several other countries where obesity is much less common than in America. So, women often weigh more in countries with more sugar in the national diet, but not always.

As we saw in chapter 2, lighter American women actually report *more* sugar calories in their diets than heavier women and most other studies also show this pattern. However, a few studies that use chemical methods to monitor sugar intake, such as measuring sugar by-products in the urine, have found somewhat higher intakes in heavier women. And some studies suggest that having more sugar-sweetened beverages, often consumed between meals, might be linked to higher weights. Heavier American women get more of their sugar than lighter women from fast foods, snacks, ice cream, pancakes or waffles, and beverages separate from meals, including soft drinks and fruit drinks, and less from milk.

Since sugar eaten between meals in beverages or snacks is linked to heavier weights, this suggests that *when* we eat sugar may make a difference. Just as having alcohol on an empty stomach increases its effects, the same may be true of sugar. When doctors test someone for diabetes, they give the patient a sugar drink to take on an empty stomach so that their blood sugar and insulin will go as high as possible. Taken with other food, it would have much less effect. Since insulin promotes fat storage, it may be best to eat sugar with other foods, for example, in desserts at the end of a meal, rather than in snacks or beverages between meals. Also, using small amounts of sugar to enhance the flavor of foods is much better than adding oils high in omega-6.

Since artificial sweeteners have very few calories, it would seem that substituting them for sugar would help keep weights down. Unfortunately, there is little evidence that women who use these sweeteners eat fewer calories or weigh less. Lighter women use much less artificial sweetener than heavier women. And while heavier women have many more sugar-free beverages than lighter women, they also have more sugar beverages. A number of studies have shown that women who use artificial sweeteners tend to gain more weight over time than those who do not. Because they fail to provide energy along with sweetness, they may increase our appetite for foods that have calories. Trying to fool Mother Nature is not always a good strategy.

Starches

In addition to simple sugars, carbohydrates include the long chains of sugars that form starches, the "complex" carbs that many nutritionists like. Ultimately, it all turns into sugar in our body, but starches take more time to digest and usually come bundled with other nutrients and fiber. Since the agricultural revolution some ten thousand years ago, starches from grains like wheat, rice, and corn and from roots like potatoes, cassava, sweet potatoes, and yams have been the major sources of calories in our diets. Our hunter-gatherer forebears probably also dug up roots and had diets moderately high in starches. Worldwide today almost two-thirds of all calories come from carbs, with more than half from starches. Americans get about a third of their calories from starches, and Europeans a bit more.

Most nutritionists would like us to eat more starches. One reason for that is Keys's idea that we should reduce our share of calories from fat, which means that we need more starch to make up for those lost fat calories. This is why the "food pyramid" has a broad base of starches. Starches generally do not seem to increase weight. Women tend to weigh less in countries with a larger share of calories from starches, as in Europe, and thinner American women tend to have more starches in their diets than heavier women. However, as we have seen, many American foods that are rich in starches are also high in omega-6, like potato chips, french fries, and many baked goods. If we can increase the calorie share of starches in our diet without increasing omega-6, it may be beneficial. Potatoes, pasta, and rice without added fat are low in omega-6 and can be eaten without restriction.

Recently, some have argued that starches are bad rather than good. Because diets very low in carbs and very high in fat, like the Atkins diet, can help some people to temporarily lose weight, this gives rise to the idea that low-carb diets are good diets and that excess weight and obesity are due to eating too many carbs. Unfortunately, low-carb diets have not proven to be any better than other diets when it comes to maintaining a lower weight. And, as we have seen, women tend to weigh less when they have more starches in their diets. Women in countries with the lowest average weights have the highest proportion of carbs in their diets. Also, carbs were not increasing in the American diet over the past forty years as our weight went up. There were much more carbs in the American diet in 1910 than there are today.

In a high-fat, low-carb diet, most of the calories come from fat, which is also what happens when we have to live off our stored fat because of a shortage of calories. When fat is broken down to use for energy, it produces ketones rather than sugars; and a high level of ketones in our blood can reduce appetite. But it's hard to argue that starvation is a normal or healthy mode of life. Except for people living in the Arctic (who are not usually thin), every normal human diet that we know of draws a major share of its calories from carbohydrates.

A related concern about the connection between certain starches and weight focuses on their "glycemic index," the effect of starches like white rice and potatoes in increasing blood sugar and insulin levels more than whole grains. Some believe that foods with a high glycemic index are more likely to promote weight gain, but there is little evidence to support this. Rice and nonfried potatoes are not linked with higher weights in American women or women in different countries. However, foods with a lower index, like whole grains, usually have more beneficial fiber.

A natural human diet has a wide variety of foods, including plenty of different vegetables and fruits, starches, and moderate amounts of meat and fish; we have evolved to be omnivores. Lighter American women tend to have a greater variety of foods in their diets than heavier women. Any diet that restricts large groups of foods is unlikely to be favorable. The best plan is to eat a diet that you find natural, comfortable, satisfying, and enjoyable while avoiding unnatural omega-6 fats and maximizing omega-3, and for most of us, that involves a variety of fats, carbs, and proteins.

Nuts, Seeds, and Oils

Vegetable Oils for Cooking

Vegetable oils are pure fat, and most are high in omega-6 and low in omega-3, especially corn and soybean oils, the oils strongly linked with higher weights in American women. Excluding the good oils, flaxseed, canola, and olive oil, the vegetable oils in our diet contain *forty times* more omega-6 linoleic than omega-3 alpha-linolenic! In addition to soybean and corn oil, safflower and sunflower seed oils are high in omega-6 and have no omega-3 and cottonseed oil has very little omega-3. So keeping all these high-omega-6 oils to a minimum is very important. For this reason, it is best to avoid "vegetable oil," or any of the others high in omega-6. These high-omega-6 oils are used more frequently by heavier women.

Olive oil is low in omega-6 and very high in monounsaturated oleic acid, though it is also low in omega-3. Both olive oil and monounsaturated fat are generally linked with lower weights. Women tend to weigh less in countries with more olive oil in the diet, and studies show lower weights and less waist fat in women with more olive oil and monounsaturated fat in their diets; they are also linked with better health. Their share of our calories fell during the time we were gaining weight. So olive oil is a good choice for cooking and salads. However, canola oil is also quite high in monounsaturated oleic and is also high in omega-3.

Regular canola oil is almost one-tenth alpha-linolenic and two-thirds oleic. Canola oil is an excellent choice for cooking, baking, and use in homemade salad dressings. However, because all omega-3s tend to react with oxygen and become rancid, canola oil should be kept tightly capped and away from light; it's probably best to buy no more than a quart at a time. You should also pay close attention to the expiration date ("best when used by") on the bottle and choose a bottle that is far from its expiration date. If you use the same bottle for more than a few weeks, you may want to keep it in the refrigerator. If used for deep-frying, it is best not to reuse canola more than a few times.

Unfortunately, just as seed companies developed soybeans with very low levels of omega-3, because of the rancidity problem, they have recently done the same with canola. So you should always choose a canola oil that lists its omega-3 (alpha-linolenic) content on the label; it should have approximately 1,300 milligrams per tablespoon (about 9 percent). Because of the new forms of canola, if canola oil is listed in a processed-food product, it may no longer be the high-omega-3 type that is most valuable. Natreon and Clear Valley "high-stability" canola oils, for example, are much lower in omega-3. Any food product that sits on a shelf is unlikely to be made with regular canola oil because it will be more prone to spoil. This is why all foods enriched with omega-3 are refrigerated. So if you find a food product on the shelf that says it "may contain" canola oil, it probably doesn't have any canola oil or at least not the desirable kind with 9 percent omega-3 alpha-linolenic.

Flaxseed oil is more than half alpha-linolenic, but having so much makes it very prone to spoil; it should always be kept in a dark bottle and refrigerated. It does not work well for cooking, but can be used on salads. Ground flaxseeds are one-fourth alpha-linolenic and one-fourth fiber and can also be added to salads and other foods, but also need to be refrigerated. Walnuts are about one-tenth alpha-linolenic, and walnut oil has a little more. However, since canola oil has less omega-6 linoleic and more oleic than walnut oil, it is generally a better, cheaper, and much more available choice. Although EPA and DHA are the forms of omega-3 that are active in the body and are the most beneficial, a diet high in omega-3 alpha-linolenic is also desirable to help keep omega-6 in check.

Salad Dressings: Make Your Own

Salad dressings made with vegetable oil (usually soybean oil) are as much as one-third omega-6 linoleic and contribute a sixth of the total linoleic in our current diet. It's best to avoid dressings which "may contain" soybean oil. Regular mayonnaise made with soybean oil is

40 percent linoleic. Caesar, cheese, and creamy dressings also tend to be very high in linoleic and Italian or vinaigrette dressings made with soybean oil are moderately high.

To avoid linoleic in salad dressings, you can choose dressings like yogurt, fruit, and sweet and sour, which usually have less oil. Low-calorie, low-fat, and fat-free dressings also tend to be low in linoleic. Dressings made with olive oil alone, like authentic Italian or vinaigrette, have very little omega-6 and are good choices, and more of these are now appearing in supermarkets. Mayonnaise made with olive oil is much tastier than the usual kind. Better yet, by making your own dressing, you can also boost beneficial omega-3 fat by using fish, flaxseed, or canola oils. Some commercial dressings have recently appeared that claim to be made with canola oil, but make sure that it is the only oil used. Remember to refrigerate all of these good oils (and the dressings you make from them) because their valuable omega-3 is highly perishable. As the public becomes more aware of our omega imbalance, more dressings based on healthier oils are likely to be available, though they may require refrigeration, like other omega-3-enriched foods. Be sure to keep reading labels!

Margarines and Butter: Nature Knows Best

Since margarine is made from vegetable oil, usually corn or soybean oil, it is about one-fifth linoleic. "Soft" margarine-like spreads are more popular and have even more omega-6. Liquid margarines are the worst, at one-third linoleic, and heavier women use more of them. Until recently, margarines were also a major source of trans fat, and even if the label claims there are zero grams of trans fat per serving, there still may be up to a half gram. The more solid a margarine is, the more likely it is to have trans fats.

One alternative to margarine is old-fashioned butter. Like other dairy products, butter is low in omega-6, and it also provides some omega-3. Lighter American women tend to eat more butter while heavier women eat more margarine. Europeans eat much more butter than Americans, due to our misguided fear of saturated fat. The French, with an obesity rate just one-sixth of ours and a coronary disease death rate one-third of ours, eat four times as much butter as Americans. People in other European countries also tend to use more butter and to have lower coronary disease rates than Americans. Butter can also be used for cooking and gives wonderful flavor to vegetables. Some food makers now offer spreads enriched with omega-3, including DHA and alpha-linolenic, and these may be preferable to other margarines and spreads.

Nuts Are Good

Nuts are puzzling, but in a good way. Although they are often relatively high in omega-6 linoleic, they do *not* seem to encourage weight gain. Lighter American women tend to eat more nuts than heavier women, and women tend to weigh less in countries with more nuts in the national diet. Other studies also show a favorable effect of nuts on weight. There is also some evidence that nuts may be beneficial to health in other ways.

As is true for other real foods, the linoleic in nuts is a normal and natural part of the nut, and there is much less than in a concentrated vegetable oil, which has been squeezed out and chemically treated to remove color, odor, and nutrients. Nuts are also high in fiber, which may also help to lower weights. America's most popular nut, the peanut, is one-sixth omega-6 linoleic, but it is also a quarter monounsaturated, a quarter protein, and a tenth fiber, and it has a variety of vitamins and nutrients, including choline, which is good for our brains. Pecans and brazil nuts have a little more linoleic than peanuts; almonds and pistachios have less; and cashews and filberts, much less. Chestnuts are very low in linoleic. Walnuts have some linoleic but also have a large amount of omega-3 alpha-linolenic, making them best of the nuts. So despite their omega-6 content, there is no need to restrict nuts and having more may be beneficial. They may be an especially good choice for snacks, particularly if they replace high-linoleic snacks like chips.

How to Find the Hidden Linoleic on a Food Label

All processed foods must inform you about their fat content, including those provided by restaurants and fast-food vendors if you ask for them (we have included many of these on our Web site at whywomenneedfat .com). Thanks to Ancel Keys, food labels have to list the total amount of fat and how much of that total is saturated fat. Some labels now also list how much is monounsaturated or polyunsaturated fat. So how do you find the linoleic?

If the label shows the amount of polyunsaturated fat, you can assume that almost all of it is linoleic, unless it says it is enriched in omega-3 and gives specifics. If the label only shows total and saturated fat, you can subtract the amount of saturated fat from the total to give the amount of unsaturated fat. As a rule of thumb, you can assume that half to two-thirds of this unsaturated fat is linoleic unless it definitely contains olive or regular canola oil. For example, if an item has eight grams of fat and two grams of saturated fat per serving, you can assume that four of the remaining six grams are omega-6 linoleic.

The list of ingredients can also be helpful. Oils high in omega-6 linoleic include soybean, corn, safflower, sunflower seed, cottonseed, and sesame seed oil. Oils that are low in linoleic and high in omega-3 include regular canola, walnut, and flaxseed oils, although low-omega-3 canola oils are beginning to appear. Olive oil is also low in linoleic. However, some products that claim to have olive or canola oil might contain other oils as well, so always check the ingredients. Unfortunately, as we have seen, because many labels now say "may contain," a manufacturer can put canola or olive oil on the "may contain" list but never use it in the product; this is a labeling loophole that should be closed. Products that sit on a grocery shelf are unlikely to have any oils that are high in omega-3.

Omega Fats and Fast Food

Most women lead busy lives and do not always have time to prepare meals for themselves or their families. More than a quarter of the calories consumed by American women comes from meals away from home. About half of this, one-eighth of our calories, comes from fast-food vendors, and another eighth comes from restaurants, cafeterias, bars, vending machines, food carts, and the like.

So what fast-food choices are better? For beverages, milk is always a good choice. Yogurt and cheese are also low in omega-6 and higher in omega-3, as are milk shakes and soft-serve ice cream. Broiled, grilled, or roasted beef or chicken without the skin is preferable to other meat dishes or sandwiches. Other good choices include uncoated shrimp, nonfried fish (a rarity), sushi, chili, croissants, and sourdough pancakes. For other meats, chicken subs (without oily dressing), meat loaf with beef, sweet and sour pork or chicken are relatively low in linoleic but also have some omega-6 arachidonic. For many more choices, see our table "Better Fast Foods" on pages 209–11.

The Bottom Line

There are more than 3,700 calories per person per day in the American food supply, but in the seven countries within one hundred calories of our figure, the average woman weighs twenty-two pounds less than the average American woman. The main difference lies in the extraordinarily large amount of vegetable oils in our foods and the omega-6 fats they contain. Our food supply is heavily laced with harmful amounts of these omega-6 fats, both because these fats are cheap and because of the mistaken belief that they would be better for our health than saturated fats. At the same time, our foods have been drained of beneficial omega-3 fats both intentionally, because they are perishable and limit shelf life, and unintentionally, because they are simply being overwhelmed by the rising tide of competing omega-6s. This makes getting our omega fats in the right balance a difficult challenge.

Having more omega-3 is the most important way to restore this balance. Fish, seafood, and fish oil are the best food sources of weight-lowering and health-promoting omega-3s. If you don't like seafood or are concerned about its mercury content, purified fish oil in liquid or capsule form is the best choice. Having more alpha-linolenic acid is also desirable; canola, walnut, and flaxseed oils have larger amounts, as do flaxseeds and walnuts themselves. Fruits and vegetables also provide omega-3 in smaller amounts. It's also a good idea to make your own salad dressings using, olive, canola, walnut, fish, or flaxseed oil and to use canola oil for your main cooking oil.

Having less omega-6 is also very important. Foods that should be limited as much as possible include soybean, corn, safflower, and sunflower oils; most salad dressings and margarines; fat from supermarket meats and poultry; most fast foods and processed prepackaged foods; fried foods; fish and meat with batters or meat "helpers"; and most commercial baked goods made with soybean oil.

In addition to foods high in omega-3, fruits and vegetables (especially those with colored nutrients), and dairy foods such as milk and yogurt are also beneficial, along with nuts and seeds, olive oil, starches, whole grains, some dark chocolate, and eating a wide variety of unprocessed foods. There is much to be said for Michael Pollan's suggestion that we eat real foods.

Foods best used in moderation include sugar, which is best as a seasoning or in a dessert at the end of a meal, and lean meats that are broiled, baked, or grilled without added fat; chicken should always be prepared and eaten without the skin. Meats from animals that are organic, free range, or grass fed are likely to be better, as are eggs with higher amounts of omega-3.

By reducing the enormous amounts of unnatural omega-6 fats in our diet, increasing omega-3, and following our guidelines for other foods and beverages, you should be able to slowly shed at least some of the unnatural excess weight that has resulted from the misbegotten changes in our diets and, in this way, move toward your "natural" weight. In the next chapter, we will look at some other choices that may help you in this process.

CHAPTER 9

Other Ways to Help Restore Your Natural Weight

O ver the past forty years American diets have changed in many ways, but, as we have seen, the biggest and most unfortunate of these changes is the shift in our omega fat balance: We now get far too much omega-6 and far too little omega-3. This is the dietary change that seems to be propelling our recent weight gains, earning us our unenviable status as the world's fattest developed nation. Our out-of-balance omegas seem to have raised the set points for our body weights. These new, higher set points increase our appetites and consequently add pounds everywhere, especially to our middles.

Changing your diet to a more natural one is the most critical step in helping you to move toward a more natural weight. However, it's unrealistic to think that this will fix the problem overnight. The amount of omega-6 and omega-3 in our blood is not determined by just our current diets. Because there is a constant exchange of nutrients between our blood and tissues, our stored fat also plays a key role. The amount of omega fats in our stored fat reflects our long-term diet, and many years of an imbalanced diet cause the same kind of imbalance in our fat stores. Despite some trading of fats between our blood and our fat stores, the process of changing the makeup of our stored fat is slow.

This is why it is important to increase all forms of omega-3 in your diet while at the same time decreasing all types of omega-6 as much as possible. By persisting in this more natural diet over time, you should begin to *slowly* move toward your natural weight, just as Valerie Frankel did.

But there are other things besides the balance between omega-6 and omega-3 that may also influence your weight and appetite and are worth keeping in mind. These include how and when you eat, the beverages you drink, the amount that you exercise, and your reliance on processed foods. So here are several other steps you can take that may help you move steadily toward your natural weight and shape.

Eat Only Until You Are Satisfied and Then Stop

Your hypothalamus works to keep your weight the same mainly by regulating your appetite. If your weight falls below your ordained set point, your brain increases your appetite so that you tend to eat more until you have come back into balance. If your weight is higher than your set point, it makes you less hungry. But this system works properly only if you pay attention to your body's signals and limit your eating to times when you feel hungry. Because eating is usually pleasurable and often linked in our minds with other positive experiences, most of us will sometimes find ourselves eating even when we are *not* hungry, whether to relieve stress, to make ourselves feel better, or just out of habit. If you often snack when reading or watching TV, these activities are likely to make you feel like eating. If you have a late-night snack today, you may well feel like having another tomorrow. Unfortunately, when we eat without hunger these unwanted calories are more likely to be stored, since they exceed what our brains are telling us we need to balance the calories we are spending. By paying attention to your appetite and sensations of fullness and by eating only until you are satisfied, you and your brain can be on the same team.

Eating until you are satisfied works best when you take your time.

During a meal, it takes a while for the nutrients from the food you are eating to make their way into your blood, inform your brain, and give you a feeling of fullness and satisfaction. So it may be helpful to eat slowly or take some breaks to give this time to happen. Europeans tend to take much more time enjoying their meals than Americans, and this may also help them to weigh less.

Reduce Your Daily Calories
by a *Small* Amount

As we saw in chapter 7, your brain is always checking to see if your food supply is compromised, so that it views any dieting that leads to a relatively rapid and sustained weight loss as evidence that you need to eat more and get back to your set point or even higher. This is why diets almost always fail. But if you reduce your daily intake by a *small* amount, you may be able to fly under your hypothalamic radar and lose weight slowly and gradually without triggering a weight-protecting response from your brain. This may help you get down to your natural weight more quickly or even five to ten pounds lower. (There is a little wiggle room in our natural set points.) Once you are eating a natural diet and your fats are back in balance, cutting just fifty calories a day should result in a loss of five pounds over a year's time. This kind of weight loss is less dramatic than the temporary weight loss achieved with a more drastic diet but is much more likely to be permanent.

Eat Breakfast, and Avoid Snacks
After Dinner

When we eat, our meals help to set our daily biological clock cycle. If you have ever taken an airplane trip to a destination more than one or two time zones away, you have probably experienced some jet lag when you arrived and when you returned home. Once again, our old friend the hypothalamus is to blame. It uses both the pattern of light and dark *and* the timing of your meals to set your twenty-four-hour biological clock. Many of your body's key functions and activities are controlled by this clock, including the hormones and brain actions that govern your appetite, digestion, and metabolism. When you travel to a place with a different light–dark pattern and eat your meals at different times, this disrupts your usual clock cycle and often makes you feel bad until your hypothalamus adjusts to the new time. One way to adjust more quickly is to start having your meals according to the time zone you are traveling to before you arrive.

In using the timing of your meals to help set your biological clock, your hypothalamus expects that you will eat soon after waking up in the morning and that you will stop eating after dark. So it expects to receive calories in the morning and is disturbed when they don't arrive on time. And it is unprepared for those that come from a late-night snack. If you fail to eat a morning meal or you eat again after your evening meal, this can disrupt its normal rhythm and lead to an abnormal clock cycle and weight gain. Because you have bright lights on at night regardless of the time of year, your hypothalamus is already likely to be somewhat disturbed. But an abnormal meal pattern makes this much worse, and disrupting your normal clock cycle in this way can cause you to gain additional weight.

One way to avoid this is to have a regular morning meal. Less than a fifth of the calories in the average American woman's diet currently come from breakfast, and this is partly because one in five women skips it. The percentage of American women eating breakfast has been declining during the time we have been gaining weight. You might think that skipping breakfast should help you weigh less, since those are calories you won't eat, but studies have shown that women who skip a morning meal tend to eat more later in the day and are more likely to gain excess weight. Calories from a morning meal are more likely to be spent than saved, and the lack of food in the morning interferes with your natural clock cycle. Some years ago, there was a diet plan that allowed you to eat anything you want before noon and less later in the day, and some people found this effective. Of course, not everyone is hungry when they wake up, but if you don't feel hungry right away, consider having a meal later in the morning. You can take some breakfast foods with you to work and have them during a morning break. Unfortunately, fast-food breakfasts such as egg sandwiches tend to be quite high in omega-6 and are not a good choice.

Just as breakfast helps to start your daily clock cycle, your evening meal tells it to start winding down. Your body normally uses the calories you have eaten in the evening to keep it running through the night. But if you consume extra calories later, you send a conflicting signal to your brain that can disrupt your whole cycle. Those unexpected calories are also more likely to turn into fat, especially if they are high in omega-6. Studies show that those who eat late at night tend to weigh more and gain more weight than those who don't. Late-night snacks can easily become a habit, so it is best to make it a rule not to eat after your evening meal.

Try to Have Smaller Portions

Imagine you are walking into a movie theater, and they offer you a bucket of free popcorn. How much of it would you eat? In an experiment done at a Philadelphia cinema, patrons were offered either four or eight ounces of popcorn that, unknown to them, was either freshly popped or two weeks old. Those given the larger bucket of fresh popcorn ate one and a half times more than those offered a smaller bucket. Even more revealing, those given a larger container of stale popcorn ate a third more than those given a smaller portion even though they did not think that it tasted very good.

Or consider this experiment. Four people sit down at a table with a bowl of soup for each of them and eat as much from the bowl as they want. But unknown to them, some bowls are connected to a small hose and additional soup is slowly pumped in as they eat. People given these secretly replenishing bowls eat almost twice as much soup as those with ordinary bowls, though they are not aware of having any more than the others. Because the bowl does not look any bigger, they do not realize that they have eaten much more.

These are examples of many experiments showing that women eat more when they are offered larger portions in a restaurant setting, including bigger soft drinks or larger helpings of french fries, macaroni and cheese, potato chips, sandwiches, or pasta. Women given larger portion sizes typically eat 10 to 20 percent more calories at the meal. (Men eat even more.) In addition, some studies suggest that heavier women tend to regularly choose or dish out larger portion sizes for themselves.

Most of these studies only look at the effect of larger portion sizes on how much women eat during a single meal, so it is possible that they will eat less at subsequent meals in order to compensate. However, one study provided either smaller or larger portions over a four-day period and found that those offered the larger portions consumed 10 percent more calories over the four days with little evidence that they cut back in calories at later meals to make up for the larger amounts from the earlier ones.

Will (and his brother) can testify to the powerful effect of portion size on how much you eat from his childhood experiences. When he was called to dinner, the modest amounts of food already on his plate were all there was and that was it. That was all he was going to get, other than occasional visits to the corner store to buy candy with his limited funds. Not until he went to a Boy Scout summer camp in his early teens did he learn that there was such a thing as second helpings, and he soon became known as the "bottomless pit." He came home considerably heavier than when he left.

So what can you do to counteract the waist-expanding effect of larger portion sizes? Try keeping in mind that we tend to eat more when there is more on a plate. Since many of us are inclined to load up our plates when we go to an "all-you-can-eat" buffet in order to get our money's worth, it is probably best to visit such buffets infrequently or to consciously eat less over the next day or two. When you go to a restaurant where a generous helping of food is brought to you on an individual plate, you can ask for another plate and treat the first plate as if it were a platter, dishing out a smaller amount to start. This also makes sharing with others easier, and any uneaten portions can be taken home. You can use the same method when you get fast food, giving yourself a smaller portion and taking the leftovers home.

The same idea applies when you eat at home. Here, you usually control how much goes on your plate, so you can try dishing out a little less than usual and using a smaller plate, keeping in mind that you can always get more. When you are hungry, you may put more on your plate than you need to be satisfied, as in "my eyes were bigger than my stomach," so try putting a little less. When you eat convenience foods, avoid using the tray or package it comes in to eat from. Instead, put a portion of it on a plate or in a bowl and have more later if that is not enough. Trying to have a bit smaller portions is an important adjunct to the strategy of taking more time to eat—giving your food time to reach your stomach and trigger the signals that you have had enough and are satisfied.

Choose Nuts and Fruit for Snacks

About one fifth of the calories in the diet of the typical American woman comes in the form of snacks, from food eaten at other than traditional mealtimes, and many snack foods are likely to promote weight gain. If you do have snacks, one study has shown that having nuts for snacks can lower weight, while sugary snacks increase weight. Since fruits are also linked with lower weights, they are also a good choice.

While frequent snacking between big meals is probably not helpful, some women prefer to eat a larger number of small meals rather than the customary three big meals. This pattern, perhaps more like that of our hunter-gatherer ancestors, does not seem to cause greater weight gain and may even be beneficial. If this seems more natural to you, it may be a better way to eat as long as you are eating the right foods and avoiding the wide array of unhealthy snack foods.

Limit Commercial Beverages

Most beverages other than water, milk, pure fruit juice, and hot tea are linked with higher weights. Compared with heavier American women, lighter women drink more milk and hot tea and similar amounts of water, regular coffee, and real fruit juice; but they have less of most other beverages. Heavier women drink more soft drinks and many more diet soft drinks, averaging ten ounces of soft drinks a day. They also have more fruit juice drinks, iced tea, tea with sweeteners, and fancier coffee drinks. Heavier women get almost a third of their sugar from these kinds of drinks, a larger share than lighter women. And as we have seen, the artificial sweeteners used in diet drinks also seem to promote weight gain.

Because sweetened soft drinks and fruit drinks provide so much of our sugar—mostly in the form of corn syrup—it's like we're having a diabetes test every day. Among eighteen countries with data on soft drinks, the United States, at fifty-seven gallons per person each year, has almost twice as much as the next country; and women weigh more in the countries with higher amounts. Since our bodies require a good deal of water, if soft drinks are readily available, it is easy to get into the habit of getting a large share of your water in that form. However, because all soft drink makers add salt to their products, in addition to sweeteners, soft drinks actually increase our need for water.

Cutting out soft drinks will eliminate the sugar that is most likely to stimulate fat storage because of its effect on our insulin. The average adult American woman has twenty-two teaspoons of sugar a day, and six of those—more than a fourth—come from sugar-sweetened beverages. By cutting those out of your diet, you can use that sugar for seasoning, chocolate, and desserts, where it is less likely to promote weight gain. You can also save a few of those calories to help achieve the kind of small daily reduction that will not trigger a reaction from your hypothalamus.

Water is the ideal noncaloric drink. It is, after all, the beverage we have evolved to drink. According to the Institute of Medicine, drinking nine cups of water per day is an "adequate" amount for adult women, while pregnant women and nursing women may need more. Municipal tap water is as good or better than bottled water in most cities and towns, and it generates a lot less trash. You can also use water filters if you are concerned about quality. But keep in mind that most of the water used by beverage makers is probably not much different from the water that comes out of your faucet. Many diets recommend drinking plenty of water, and many women consciously drink more water to help them lose weight. Some studies support the idea that drinking more water, especially before a meal, may help to prevent weight gain, and since water is good for health, having several glasses a day seems like a good idea.

We also have some evidence that modest amounts of alcohol may also be beneficial for women's weights, especially wine. Europeans, weighing much less than we do, have a somewhat larger share of calories from alcohol than Americans and, notably, drink *four times* more wine. This suggests that wine can help to moderate weight, and women weigh less in countries with more wine in the diet. Lighter American women average *twice* as much wine as heavier women. Other studies have also shown lower weights with modest amounts of alcohol in the diet and that wine has the most benefit. Modest amounts of alcohol can also raise the level of good cholesterol (HDL) in the blood and may have other health benefits. One study suggests that the health benefit of having moderate amounts of alcohol may come from increasing omega-3 levels in the blood. So, a glass or two of wine a day—but not much more—may be helpful in keeping weight down as well as helping your heart.

Get Regular Exercise

Although our brains usually adjust our intake of calories to match the amount we are spending, regular moderate exercise may help you to have a more natural weight. Americans walk less than the slimmer Australians and Swiss, and weights tend to be lower in countries where people take more trips by bicycle or on foot and in American cities and states where more people commute to work by cycling or walking. Only one American woman in twelve walks for at least thirty minutes a day, the amount considered to be the minimum necessary for good health. Pedometer records show that lower-weight American women take twice as many steps a day as heavier women.

Some 35 million American women, about two-thirds of those who tried to lose weight in the past year, have increased the amount they exercise to help them lose weight. On average, they gained a half pound less weight by year's end than those who did not try to exercise more. Looking back, the exercisers have also gained a bit less weight in the past ten years. Moderate exercise by itself is not likely to be enough to move women back to their natural weights, but it may help when combined with a change to a more natural diet.

Lighter American women are almost twice as likely as heavier women to engage in vigorous exercise (running, swimming, cycling) and even more likely to exercise using weights. They also spend fewer hours watching TV and burn almost twice as many calories in their leisure activities. However, since arthritis is more common in obese women, some of them may be less active because activity is more difficult and painful; so it is not easy to determine whether less exercise is a cause or a result of obesity. As noted in chapter 6, it is clear that obese women who do exercise regularly have much lower health risks than those who do not.

Since walking and other forms of moderate exercise are unquestionably beneficial for health, there are very good reasons to be active at any weight. Walking for an additional twenty to thirty minutes a day would be a good start for many of us, and wearing a pedometer to keep track of your steps is often helpful. One study found that overweight women who walked ten thousand steps a day lost an average of five pounds over nine months; this should also have health benefits. Lifting some weights while watching TV could help turn a bad habit into a good one. Combined with a more natural diet, moderate daily exercise may help a woman to find her natural healthy weight.

Reduce the Amount of Processed Food in Your Diet

In addition to eating more of our meals outside the home, another major reason for America's rising weights is that even at home we eat more processed and prepared foods, foods that are generally high in omega-6 and low in omega-3. According to annual surveys of American eating patterns, almost half of the main dishes we now serve at dinner are ready-to-eat or frozen prepared foods; just thirty years ago, in 1980, three-quarters of our main dishes were made from scratch.

One disturbing study highlights the large share of prepared foods in the diets of today's young adult women (a group who are much heavier than in the past). The authors looked at how often young adult women aged eighteen to twenty-three prepare their own meals. Only one in three bought fresh vegetables or had a green salad at least once a week, and less than one in four prepared at least one meal a week with chicken, fish, or vegetables. Lack of time was a factor for some of these women; about two-fifths said they did not have enough time to prepare meals. But many of the women who did not feel that time was a problem were also basing their diets on prepared foods.

Some people may be less inclined to have real foods because they think these foods cost more, but this is simply incorrect. Unprocessed foods are actually substantially cheaper. Not surprisingly, processing foods costs more than not processing them. Raw vegetables will obviously cost less to produce than a similar amount of a frozen precooked and preseasoned vegetable dish with added vegetable oil. One recent study found that the cost per calorie in a diet of convenience foods was one-fourth higher than in a diet of healthy whole foods despite the high level of inexpensive calorie-rich sugar and fat in convenience foods.

Perhaps surprisingly, surveys find that most of those who rely on convenience foods agree that they cost more, are less healthy, and do not taste as good as real foods; and most say they would enjoy cooking if they had more time. This suggests that most American women are well aware that meals based on processed convenience foods are less healthy and less desirable than meals in which fresh or frozen raw ingredients are used to prepare a meal. Yet despite this understanding, a large portion of our diets is still based on these expensive and unhealthy foods. The main reason for this seems to be a lack of time for preparing meals.

So understanding that limitations in time are a serious problem, what can you do to increase the amount of real food in your diet and decrease the amount of processed food? Is it possible to cook meals at home with real food without taking a large amount of time? Yes. There are several options you can consider that allow you to prepare quick and easy meals with real food ingredients.

One method of cooking real food quickly is stir-frying. While this does use a small amount of oil, healthful canola oil works fine. In stir-frying, you can quickly cook small pieces of fish or meat such as chicken, pork, or beef together with a vegetable like bell peppers, snow peas, green beans, broccoli, onions, or asparagus. Typical seasonings include soy sauce, garlic, ginger, and chilies. Stir-fries are usually eaten with rice, and an automatic rice cooker can make rice preparation quick and easy as well. Similar kinds of quick meals can be made with whole-grain noodles. If you make extra amounts, they can be reheated in a microwave for an even quicker meal at a later time. There are many books on fast and easy stir-fries, including those by Helen Chen, Ken Hom, Susan Jane Cheney, Carol Palmer, and Martin Yan, and many Web sites that provide recipes and show how to do it.

Another cooking method that can save personal time is using a slow cooker. You can put food in late at night or first thing in the morning and have it cook for six or eight hours at low heat while you sleep or work, resulting in very tender meats. There are many cookbooks on slow-cooker meals, and also on one-pot or one-dish meals. Grilling is also a relatively quick and beneficial way to cook meats or vegetables. There are a great many cookbooks that feature quick and easy meal preparation.

Another option to consider is to cook enough for the whole week on one day when you have more time available. This idea has been developed by Rachael Ray in her *Week in a Day* program on the Cooking Channel, and many of her recipes are also available online. If moving to real foods all at once is too big a step, consider some hybrid meals as a transition, using both real and processed foods. Sandra Lee's "semi-homemade" cooking is an example of this approach. However, it's important to use processed foods that are low in added vegetable fats by following the suggestions in the last chapter.

Putting It All Together

The best way to find your natural weight is to return to a more natural and healthy diet high in omega-3 and low in omega-6 and to link this fat-rebalancing strategy with some of the other steps we have suggested. Unlike the thrill of losing several pounds in a matter of days, only to have them come back weeks later, the weight loss that comes from this approach will be gradual but *lasting*. With this kind of slow-paced program, it may be best not to weigh yourself frequently, but to just concentrate on doing the right things. You should find that having a more natural diet together with a moderate amount of physical activity is more satisfying and more conducive to positive feelings than the usual American diet. Your goal should be to adopt a way of eating that is balanced, healthy, satisfying, and sustainable and which, like virtue, is its own reward. If you follow these principles, your weight should take care of itself. It may not be the body of your dreams, but, hopefully, it will be more like the one you were meant to have and one that can give you years of better health and satisfaction. In the next chapter, we will look at how you can get a better idea of what kind of body you were meant to have.

CHAPTER 10

Finding Your Natural Weight and Body Type

In one of the saddest studies we know of, researchers from Yale University recently set up a Web site and invited visitors to express their opinions about weight. More than four thousand responded, and more than 80 percent were women. A large majority of those who responded were overweight or obese, just like two-thirds of American women. But most still said they preferred "thin people" to "fat people." And almost a third of those who were heavy also agreed with the statement that "fat people" are less motivated and lazier than thinner people.

Even more disturbing were people's responses when asked what kinds of terrible things they would be willing to suffer rather than be obese. Almost half said they would be willing to give up a year of life rather than be obese, and one in six said they would give up *ten* years of life. One in three said they would rather be divorced, and one in four said they would rather be unable to have children. Nearly one in ten said they would rather have a child with a learning disability than one who was obese. And one in twenty said they would rather lose an arm or leg or be blind than be obese.

These results are unfortunate, even tragic, because they are based on the faulty assumption that our differences in weight depend largely on what we do. But, as we have seen, weight is much less modifiable than most people think. By using twin studies and comparisons among relatives, we can tell that our weight is largely set by our genes: Roughly 65 to 70 percent of the differences in weight between people are associated with the particular genes they happen to have, making it extremely difficult for a naturally heavy person to be thin. Genes are especially influential in setting your lowest possible weight and in limiting how much weight you can lose.

At the moment you are conceived, you are entered into a gene lottery when your mother's and father's genes pair up for the first time. Each provides a unique mix of the genes that came from your grandparents, as the two copies of each of your parent's twenty-three chromosomes are randomly sliced, diced, and reassembled into a single set. Some of us will happen to get a mix of genes that will make us lighter than average, but some of us will inevitably receive a mix that makes us heavier. No one is to blame for this; it is simply the luck of the draw after the shuffle of the genetic deck that dictates whether you will be very thin, very heavy, or in between.

But while our genes have not changed, the unnatural changes in the American diet over the past fifty years have made almost all American women heavier than they would have otherwise been. These dietary changes have distorted the intent of our genes and made it more difficult for us to know how heavy we would have been if we were still eating a more natural diet.

Inside most of us is a thinner person with the "natural weight" that we would have had were it not for these recent unfortunate dietary changes. Reversing those dietary changes should help to reverse the changes they have caused in our bodies. By eating a more natural, omega-balanced diet, we should be able to gradually reverse at least some of this excess weight gain and move back toward our natural weights, as we saw in chapter 7 with the stories of Valerie Frankel, Graziella, and Joanna.

The best way to discover your natural weight is to return to a natural diet. If you follow the recommendations we have made in the past two chapters, you should gradually move back toward your natural weight and body shape. Remember that this weight is not a goal you should strive for; it is what you can expect to happen naturally—without counting or restricting your calories and without feeling hungry—if you bring your omega-6 and omega-3 fats into balance and follow the other simple recommendations in the last two chapters. But there is a way you can get an idea right now of the weight and body type nature intended for you, as we will now see.

What Girls (and Women) Are Made Of

Laurie and Melanie are both in their late twenties and each stands five feet, four inches tall, weighs 140 pounds, and has a BMI of 24. Since all of these measurements are the same, you might suppose that their bodies would be quite similar. Yet, even though they match on all three, the nature of their weight and their body type is quite different. If they step onto the metal bars of an electronic scale designed to estimate percentage of body fat, we can see where one difference lies. Of Laurie's 140 pounds, 29 percent, or 40 pounds, is fat, while Melanie has 39 percent, or 55 pounds, of fat. Melanie has 15 more pounds of fat than Laurie, and Laurie has 15 more pounds of lean nonfat tissue than Melanie. Because Laurie's extra lean tissue balances Melanie's added fat, they happen to weigh the same. The amount and proportion of muscle and fat in a woman's body has a very big effect on how much she weighs and on her natural weight and body type.

Every woman's weight is the result of her unique mixture of bone, muscle, organs, and fat. The way these factors combine together determines her body's size, shape, and total weight. Each of these can vary separately from the others, though bones, muscles, and organs tend to go together, and each is strongly influenced by her particular mix of genes. Women whose genes give them bigger bones need more muscle to move and support them: Each pound of bone requires about ten pounds of muscle. And women with more bone and muscle require bigger organs to control and nourish them and more supporting tissues. Each pound of muscle requires about a pound of other lean tissue. (Fat requires much less.) So let's see now just how your bones, muscle, and fat each contribute to your natural weight.

Bone and Muscle

The effect of a woman's bones on her weight was first explored by Louis Dublin, a statistical expert at the Metropolitan Insurance Company. He was trying to figure out what weights make men or women healthy or unhealthy by using the measurements and survival rates of 4 million men and women who had purchased life insurance. Dublin found that women who weighed much more than average were less healthy, but he also found that the average weight for women with the same height was different depending on what he called their "body frames." He determined the size of a woman's body frame from the size of her bones, such as the width of her elbow, and found that women with bigger bones weighed more. For example, he found that a woman whose elbow was just a quarter inch wider than another woman's elbow typically weighed about twenty pounds more, because her bigger bones needed more muscle, bigger organs, and more supporting tissues. And some women's genes happen to give them bigger bones and greater muscularity.

In 1942, Dublin published his first table of "ideal body weights" with ranges of recommended weights for men and women of different heights and for three types of "body frame": small, medium, and large. For most heights, the table allowed a woman with a "large frame" to weigh ten pounds more than a woman with a "medium frame" and twenty pounds more than a woman with a "small frame" and still be considered "healthy" for insurance purposes. Women who weighed more than the average for their body frame had more fat. Dublin's tables, which were updated periodically, became the standard way for deciding whether someone's weight was healthy until the 1980s, when Ancel Keys suggested that calculating the body mass index was simpler.

Dublin's work shows that in addition to your height, your natural weight also strongly depends on your bones and muscle.

Taller women have longer bones in their legs, hip, and spine than shorter women, and these longer bones require more muscle and support. Being an inch taller or shorter generally increases or decreases your weight by about five pounds. The heights of a representative group of adult American women range from forty-eight to seventy-four inches, a difference of more than two feet. When people have enough to eat, about four-fifths of those differences are determined by the genes they inherit from their parents.

A woman's height also affects her body's shape. Taller women tend to have narrower waists, shoulders, and hips in relation to their height than shorter women, and this makes them appear slimmer. They can afford to have narrower waists, for example, because they have more room between their ribs and the hips, and this is one reason that Playmates have such small waists. Because most models are very tall, this makes them seem slimmer.

Women of the same height also vary in how thick their bones are, which is also largely determined by their genes. As Dublin found, one good indication of the size of your bones is the width of your elbow and wrist. The wrist of the average American woman is two inches wide and her elbow is two and a half inches wide, but they can vary by as much as two inches. One reason that Laurie has more lean tissue than Melanie is that she has thicker bones and a wider wrist and elbow, and her thicker bones require more muscle. Quite small differences in the thickness of these joints are connected with big differences in the amount of muscle and weight.

The length of your bones determines not only your height but also how wide, broad, or "stocky" your body is. This can be seen in the width of your shoulders and hip bones (pelvis) and is also strongly determined by your genes. Women of the same height can have a broader or narrower body width. Laurie's shoulders, for example, are more than a half inch wider than Melanie's, and her hips are three-quarters of an inch wider. For the average adult American woman, shoulder width is fifteen inches and hip width is eleven inches, and both increase with height.

Women with wider bodies, like Laurie, also usually have more muscle, so the size of your bones and the breadth of your body both determine how muscular you are likely to be. Because Laurie's thicker bones and wider hips and shoulders require more muscle and bigger organs than Melanie's, she has fifteen pounds more of nonfat weight. The average American woman has about twenty pounds of bone, forty-nine pounds of muscle, and twenty-eight pounds of organs and support tissues in addition to her sixty-eight pounds of fat. Of course, women who use their muscles more also have larger muscles than those who use them less.

Body Fat

In addition to differences in muscle and bone, women's bodies also vary in how much fat they have and where it is located. Laurie not only has more muscle than Melanie, she also has less fat; but they weigh the same because the two happen to balance each other out. In a representative group of American women today, the amount of fat ranges from eighteen to more than two hundred pounds; the average percentage of fat is 41 and varies from 18 to 60 percent. As you might guess, how much fat you have is also strongly governed by your genes. Even when women have the same BMI, like Laurie and Melanie, their fat can differ by 10 to 25 percent, depending on their height.

The changes in the American diet that have led to our increased weights have not only added pounds, but they appear to have also increased the proportion of our weight that is fat. When we compare the percentage of body fat in today's American women with other groups of women with similar BMIs, American women seem to have more fat. We not only weigh more, but more of our weight is fat. Returning to a more natural diet should help you to lower your percentage of fat as well as your weight.

But women with the same amount of body fat can also differ in where it is located and how much they have in their waists, hips, and legs. We have seen that women tend to increase their waist fat and decrease their lower-body fat as they have children and age, but some women naturally have more of their fat in their lower body or their waist, and this, too, is strongly influenced by each woman's genes. The average waist size of a representative group of adult American women measured just above the hips is thirty-seven inches and ranges from twenty-two to seventy inches, and is strongly related to a woman's overall percentage of body fat. Even for women with the same BMI, waist sizes can differ by ten to fifteen inches. For example, Laurie's waist size is twenty-five inches, seven inches smaller than Melanie's thirty-two-inch waist.

Your total weight is the sum of the weight of your bones, muscles, organs, and fat. When you gain weight, most of the added weight is fat, but it also includes some muscle and bone. On average, an increase or decrease of one pound in your weight includes ten ounces of fat and six ounces of lean tissue, including half an ounce of bone. So how much bone, muscle, and fat you have needs to be considered in order to predict what your natural weight would be if you were eating a more natural diet.

Four Steps to Estimating Your Natural Weight

The first step toward estimating your natural weight is to look at the weights of your older relatives when they were your age. The second step is to compare your current weight with other women your age and with American women from the time before the flood of omega-6 increased our weights. The third step is to see if you have more or less muscle than average by assessing the size of your bones and the width of your body. And the last step is to estimate how much fat you have and your percentage of fat based on your BMI and the size of your waist.

1. How to Find Your Natural Weight in Old Photos

Most American women today are heavier than they would have been in the past and heavier than the natural weight programmed for them by their genes. To find out what your natural weight would be, a good place to start is looking at photographs of family members who are genetically directly related to you, including your parents, grandparents, aunts and uncles, and cousins. The best photos to use are ones taken when they were about the same age as you are now and before American weights began to go up. You can also ask them to recall how much they weighed at your age. Digging out old photos of your older relatives or finding out what they weighed when younger is likely to be the most revealing since they are less likely to have been affected by the changes in the American diet over the past fifty years. There is some evidence that a woman's weight may be more influenced by her mother's genes than her father's, so you may want to pay a little more attention to your mother's side of the family.

If your blood relations were heavier or lighter than the average for their time, then it is likely that you will be, too. For example, when Graziella, the woman whose weight is now steady at 212 pounds, looked at her family photos, all of the women were quite heavy. And this is true in general: If your mother, grandmother, and other female relatives were heavier than average at your age, your own natural weight is likely to be on the heavy side no matter what kind of diet you have.

If you find that your older female relatives tended to weigh less than you when they were your age, then you are likely to be above your natural weight. Since Jessica's mother Susan weighed around 120 pounds in her early twenties and her grandmother weighed a little less, Jessica's natural weight is likely to be similar to theirs, much less than her current weight of 145 pounds. Similarly, we would expect Susan's natural weight today to be closer to 146, her mother's weight at her age, rather than her current 166.

If your weight is quite close to what your mother, grandmother, and other older female relatives weighed at your age and you are eating a natural diet, then you may already be near your natural weight. But if you are heavier than was typical for your older relatives, your natural weight is probably lower than your current weight. The more you have been exposed to the current American diet high in omega-6 fat, processed foods, fast foods, and other prepared meals, the more weight you are likely to lose by returning to a more natural diet.

2. How to Estimate Your Natural Weight from Your Current Weight

Say that we went back in time to the 1960s and carefully chose one hundred very representative American women under thirty years of age and asked them to line up according to their weight, from left to right. Each of these hundred women would be representing many thousands of women with similar weights. If we did this, the fifth woman from the left would weigh 100 pounds, the woman in the middle would weigh 126 pounds, and the ninetieth woman, way to the right, would weigh 160 pounds. And if we were to go today to a European country like Poland or Denmark and select a representative group of young women in the same way, the weight of each woman in their lines would be similar to the woman with the same position in the line of American women from the 1960s.

But if we do the same thing with a representative group of one hundred young American women today, *everyone* in today's line will be heavier. Whatever your position is in today's line, you will be heavier than the woman in the same place from the 1960s. If you are fifth in line today you will weigh 108 instead of 100 pounds; if you are in the middle, you will weigh 150 instead of 126; and if you are number ninety, you will weigh 230 pounds, *seventy* pounds more than the woman in your position from the 1960s. The further down the line you are, the more you will weigh compared with the woman in the same position in line in the 1960s. The more you would have weighed naturally without the unfortunate changes in the American diet, the more weight you are likely to have gained because of those changes.

The same kinds of differences between weights today and in the past are seen for women who are thirty or older. Once again, today's European women are quite similar in their weights to the American women from the 1960s, while each of today's American women will be heavier than her earlier counterpart. But perhaps because these somewhat older women have been less exposed to the recent dietary changes, some of the differences between the women in the two lines are smaller. Today's woman over thirty who is fifth in line weighs 113 compared with 107 in the 1960s; the woman in the middle weighs 160 compared with 140; and the ninetieth woman is 224 versus 186, a difference of thirty-eight pounds rather than seventy.

As we have explained in the earlier chapters, we believe that the reason why all of the women in today's line are heavier is that they have been eating a very different diet from the women in the 1960s or the diet eaten by European women today. But if today's American women can change to a diet more like the 1960s diet or today's European diets, their weights should *naturally* become more like the weights of the women in the same positions in line in the 1960s or in a line of European women.

Although your weight is influenced by your diet and lifestyle, your position in line today is still largely determined by your genes, so it is likely to be similar to what your position in line would have been in the 1960s. If you are near the beginning of the line today, you would likely have been in the first part of the line then. If you are heavier than average today, you would likely have been heavier than average then as well, though you would have weighed much less. So by looking at just where you are in today's line, you can see where you would have probably been in line in the 1960s. And because we can specify the weight that corresponds to each position in those lines, this can give you an indication of how much you would have weighed if you were eating an omega-balanced diet and so provide another estimate of what your natural weight would be.

The following two graphs allow you to see where you are on today's line and the corresponding point in the line of American women from the 1960s, depending on your age. This will give you a second way of estimating your natural weight, in addition to comparing yourself with your relatives when they were your age. As you will see by the way the lines become farther apart as weights go up, the more you weigh today, the farther you are likely to be from your natural weight. It's important to emphasize that these estimates apply to American women who are eating today's typical American diet. If your weight is similar to your relatives at your age and you have been eating a natural diet, you may already be at your natural weight.

Finding Your Natural Weight If You Are Under 30

Find your current weight in pounds on the left side of the graph, and use a ruler to draw a horizontal line from your weight until it crosses the solid "weight now" line, and mark that point. Then draw a vertical line down to see where it crosses the dotted "natural weight" line, and

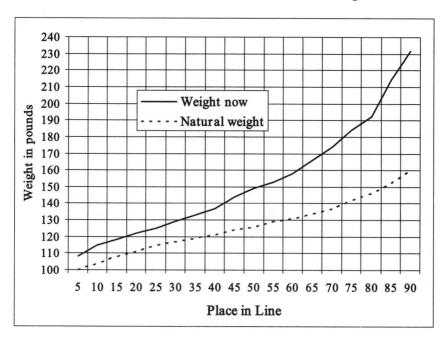

this will be your natural weight. For example, if you weigh 150 pounds, that intersection will be halfway across the "weight now" line, near the 50th position, and the corresponding weight below this weight on the dotted line would be 127 pounds, your natural weight. If you weigh more than 230 pounds, subtract 90 pounds from your current weight to get your natural weight.

FINDING YOUR NATURAL WEIGHT IF YOU ARE 30 OR OLDER

Find your current weight in pounds on the left side of the graph, and use a ruler to draw a horizontal line from your weight until it crosses the solid "weight now" line, and mark that point. Then draw a vertical line down from that point to see where it crosses the dotted "natural weight" line, and this will be your natural weight. For example, if you weigh 160 pounds, that intersection would be halfway across the "weight now" line, near the 50th position. Then look for the corresponding weight below that weight on the dotted "natural weight"

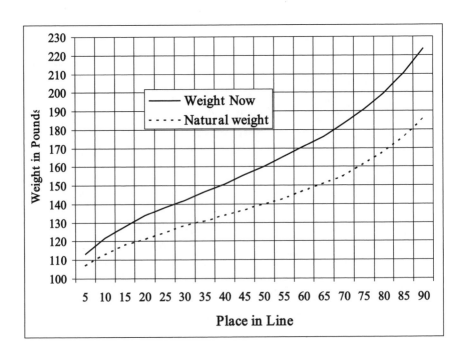

line, which would be 140 pounds for someone now weighing 160. If you weigh more than 230 pounds, subtract 50 pounds from your current weight to get your natural weight.

ESTIMATING YOUR NATURAL BMI

You can use a similar procedure to let you see what your natural BMI would be. The table below uses the same kind of comparison to give you an idea of your natural BMI—what your BMI would be if you had been eating a more natural diet with a proper balance of omega fats, like the American diet of the 1960s or European diets of today.

Your Natural BMI

First calculate your current BMI: Multiply your weight in pounds by 703 (weight × 703). Multiply your height in inches by itself (height × height). Now divide your "weight" number by your "height" number. This is your current BMI.

Your Current BMI	Your Natural BMI	
	Under Age 30	Age 30+
16	15	15
17	15	16
18	16	17
19	16	18
20	17	18
21	18	20
22	19	21
23	20	22
24	20	22
25	21	23
26	22	24
27	22	24
28	23	25
29	23	26

30	24	27
31	25	28
32	25	29
33	26	30
34	26	31
35	27	31
36	28	32
37	29	33
38	29	34
39	30	35
40	30	35
41	31	36
42	32	37
43	34	38
44	35	39
45	36	40

3. How to Estimate Your Body Type from Your Bone and Body Widths

Finding your position in line as a guide to what your natural weight and BMI would be gives you an approximate estimate for your overall weight. But your natural weight will also be affected by your particular body type. As we have seen, women with bigger bones need more muscle and will weigh more than those who have less. So if you have bigger and wider bones than average, your natural weight will be higher than the one estimated from average women. You can do an approximate assessment of your body type to see how you compare with the average, using a tape measure, yardstick, and a ruler with a centimeter scale. The larger your measurements are compared with the average, the more bone and muscle you will have, and the more you will naturally weigh. Measuring some of these is easier if you have a friend to help you.

Keep in mind that these measurements are usually made by people with special training using instruments designed for this purpose, and you may be able to have them done in this way at a fitness or exercise club. We will show you how to make approximate measurements, but they will not be very precise. However, since there are four different widths you can measure, you can compare the four with each other. If all of them seem to be higher or lower than the average, then that indicates your muscle weight is also likely to be more or less than average.

Measuring Your Elbow and Wrist Width

Louis Dublin used the width of the elbow to help determine a woman's "body frame," and the width of your wrist also indicates the general thickness of your bones. So measuring your elbow and wrist width is one way to estimate your muscularity. In both cases, you want to measure the widest distance between the outer edges of the bones. To do this, you need to press hard to squeeze out the softer tissues, such as blood vessels and fat. For your elbow, you measure the widest width of the end of the upper arm bone, which lies at the back of your elbow. For your wrist, it is the distance between the outside of the bones in the widest part of the wrist above your hand with your palm turned down. To approximate the width, you can put your thumb on one side and your index or second finger on the other, pressing firmly against the bony part, and then keep them separated by that amount as you move them over to a ruler to measure how far apart they are. You can also mark the skin at the places where you feel the bone and measure the distance between the marks. For the wrist measurement, you can also place your hand on a piece of paper, mark the sides of your wrist bones on the paper, and then measure the distance between the marks. Because the metric scale is better for measuring small distances, a ruler divided into centimeters and millimeters is more useful for this type of measurement. (Plastic rulers usually have inches on one side and centimeters and millimeters on the other.) Measuring several times may help to reduce errors.

In a representative group of American women, the average elbow when measured in this way is 6.5 centimeters wide (65 millimeters), or two and a half inches; the average wrist is 5.2 centimeters wide (52 millimeters), or about two inches. Since Laurie and Melanie are of average height, these are also the average values that apply to them. However, these widths naturally vary with one's height because taller women tend to have wider joints. Using the "Average Bone Widths" table on page 186, you can find the average measurement for women with your height. If you have wider-than-average joints, you are likely to have more muscle and be heavier. Just a small difference increases weight by a lot: A one-millimeter increase in the width of the elbow or wrist increases your natural weight by about five pounds. So for every millimeter that either of your widths is higher or lower than the average for your height, you add or subtract five pounds from your estimated natural weight.

MEASURING YOUR SHOULDER WIDTH (BIACROMIAL BREADTH)

Differences in the width, breadth, or "stockiness" of women's bodies are reflected in the width of their shoulders and hips, and women whose shoulders and hips are wider than average will also tend to have more muscle and weigh more. Women with wider elbows and wrists usually have wider body builds as well, though this is not always true.

To measure the width of your shoulders, you start by feeling along the top of your shoulder. You are feeling for the outside of the bony protrusion where your shoulder blade meets your collarbone; this is called the acromion. It may help if you look at some pictures of the acromion on the Internet. You can also start on the side of your shoulder and move up until you come to this bone, or feel along your shoulder blade in back or along your collarbone in front until you come to it.

The acromion is separate from the top of your upper arm (humerus) and does not change position when you move your upper arm. Your shoulder width is the distance from the outside border of the acromion of one shoulder to the outside of the other. If you make a mark on the outside of each one, you can use a tape measure or yardstick to measure the distance between them in inches, though it will probably be easier for someone else to measure for you. (You could also try measuring in front of a mirror.)

The shoulder width for a typical adult American woman is about fifteen inches, and the average value also increases as height goes up. You can use the "Average Bone Widths" table on page 186 to see what the average shoulder width is for a woman with your height. If your width is greater than that average, you will usually have more muscle and therefore more weight for your height. A small difference in your shoulder width has a much greater impact on your weight than the same difference in your height. For women of the same height, an increase of a quarter of an inch in shoulder width is linked to a six-pound increase in weight, so if your measurement is above or below average you can add or subtract accordingly.

MEASURING YOUR HIP WIDTH (BIILIAC BREADTH)

The last way to see how your body frame compares with other women is to measure the distance between the outside edges of your hip bone (ilium), the widest part of your pelvis. You start by feeling down along your side until you come to the top of your hip bone on each side, move around to the outside edge, and mark it. It may help to look at some pictures of the pelvis and "iliac crest" on the Internet. You then pass a tape measure or yardstick from one mark to the other while keeping it straight, even if it indents your belly, and measure the distance in inches. The average width for American women is eleven inches, but it also varies with one's height. You can compare the width of your hips with the average for your height by using the "Average Bone Widths" table on page 186. When height is the same, a quarter-inch difference in the width of your hips leads to a five-pound difference in your weight.

Average Bone Widths for Women of Different Heights

Women who are taller than seventy inches or shorter than fifty-eight inches should add or subtract 0.1 units for each of the four averages for each inch that they are taller or shorter.

Your Height	Average Measurement			
	Shoulder Width	Hip Width	Elbow Width	Wrist Width
INCHES	INCHES	INCHES	CENTIMETERS	CENTIMETERS
58	13.7	11.1	6.2	5.0
59	13.9	11.1	6.3	5.0
60	14.0	11.2	6.3	5.1
61	14.1	11.3	6.4	5.1
62	14.3	11.4	6.4	5.1
63	14.4	11.4	6.5	5.2
64	14.6	11.5	6.5	5.2
65	14.6	11.5	6.5	5.2
66	14.8	11.6	6.6	5.2
67	14.9	11.7	6.6	5.3
68	15.1	11.8	6.7	5.3
69	15.2	11.8	6.7	5.4
70	15.4	11.9	6.8	5.4

USING THE FOUR MEASUREMENTS TO ESTIMATE YOUR BODY TYPE

By comparing your shoulder, hip, elbow, and wrist widths to the averages for your height, you can see whether your bone widths are smaller or larger than average. If they are smaller, you will need less muscle and weigh less; if larger, you will need more muscle and would expect to weigh more than the average for your height, regardless of how much fat you have, just as Dublin's three types of body frame showed. You can determine whether you should add or subtract weight for each of these four measurements, and average the predicted changes to see whether your bone and muscle increases or decreases your estimated natural weight. If your muscle weight is higher or lower than average, you should also adjust your estimated natural BMI by one unit for every five pounds. Let's see how this applies to Laurie and Melanie.

Laurie's and Melanie's Bone Measurements

	Measurements		Average for 64-Inch Height (from Table)	Weight Adjustment	Change in Pounds	
	LAURIE	MELANIE			LAURIE	MELANIE
Elbow (mm)	67	64	65 mm	1 mm = 5 lbs.	+10	−5
Wrist (mm)	54	51	52 mm	1 mm = 5 lbs.	+10	−5
Shoulder (in.)	15	14.4	14.6 in.	1 inch = 24 lbs.	+10	−5
Hips (in.)	12	11.25	11.5 in.	1 inch = 20 lbs.	+10	−5
			Sum		+40	−20
			Average = Sum divided by 4		+10	−5

The table above has the measurements for Laurie and Melanie. Since Laurie's elbow is 67 millimeters, compared with 65 for the average value, her extra two millimeters equals ten extra pounds. Since Melanie's elbow is 64, or one millimeter less than the average, that is a deduction of five pounds. The other three measurements show similar differences between them, and the average of all four shows that Laurie should weigh about ten pounds more than average and Melanie should weigh about five pounds less than average.

If Laurie were estimating her natural weight, she would start with the estimate of her natural weight based on her place in today's line and add ten pounds to the estimate based on average women, while Melanie would subtract five pounds from her estimate. Taken together, these measurements predict a fifteen-pound difference between Laurie and Melanie, and we find this same fifteen-pound difference in their lean nonfat weights. At the end of the chapter is a worksheet so you can make this same calculation for yourself.

4. How to Estimate Your Body Fat

Estimating your body fat is a two-step process. The first step is to see what the average percentage of body fat is for someone with your BMI. The second step is to measure your waist size to see what percentage of fat it indicates. If your waist size is larger or smaller than average, you will have a higher or lower percentage of fat than your BMI predicts.

FINDING THE AVERAGE PERCENTAGE OF FAT FOR YOUR BMI

Generally, a one-unit increase in BMI increases fat by 1 to 2 percent. For women over fifty, the percentage of fat tends to be about 4 percent higher for a given BMI than for women who are still having their periods, as some of the muscle of older women is often replaced by fat. To see the predicted percentage of fat for your BMI and age group, find your BMI on the following "Estimating Your Body Fat" table.

Your percentage of fat is also influenced by how much you exercise, since exercise increases the size of your muscles regardless of your natural muscularity. If two women have the same BMI and one exercises more than the other, she will usually have more muscle and a lower percentage of fat. If you engage in strenuous exercise on a regular basis, such as running, rowing, biking, or team sports, subtract two percent from the body fat percentage indicated for your BMI. Weight training to strengthen muscles also tends to lower the percentage of fat. If you do regular muscle building with free weights or weight machines subtract another two percent. If you do both, subtract four percent. Unfortunately, vigorous exercise does not guarantee that you will have a low body fat; half of American women who exercise vigorously still have 40 percent or more body fat.

Estimating Your Body Fat (Amount and Percentage) from Your BMI

For higher BMIs, add a half percent to the percentage of body fat for each one-unit increase in BMI.

Your Current BMI	Your Estimated:		
	Body Fat, in Pounds	Percentage of Body Fat, for Ages:	
		18–49	50+
18	32	28	30
19	35	30	31
20	39	32	33
21	42	32	35
22	46	34	38
23	50	35	39
24	54	36	40
25	59	38	41
26	63	39	42
27	65	39	42
28	69	41	43
29	74	42	44
30	78	43	44
31	80	43	45
32	82	44	45
33	87	44	46
34	93	45	46
35	96	45	46
36	96	46	47
37	103	46	47
38	107	47	48
39	113	47	48
40	115	48	49
41	122	48	49
42	126	49	50

43	128	49	50
44	131	50	51
45	131	50	51

USING YOUR WAIST SIZE TO ESTIMATE YOUR PERCENTAGE OF FAT

If Laurie and Melanie use only their BMIs to estimate their percentage of fat, both women's BMI of 24 predicts 36 percent fat, but we know that Laurie has 29 percent fat and Melanie has 39 percent. The reason that both women's percentages of fat are different from the average for their height is that they have different amounts of fat in their waists and different waist sizes. If Laurie had the same waist size as Melanie instead of being seven inches smaller, she would have much more fat in her body and would weigh more than Melanie. So to get a better idea of your percentage of fat, you need to use your waist size as well as your BMI.

Waist size can be measured in several different ways. Models measure their minimal waist circumference, the smallest waist between their hips and ribs. Doctors, on the other hand, measure the waist just above the hips, sometimes called the "trouser waist," and this is the measurement you can use to compare yourself with other American women. The trouser waist tends to be about three inches larger than the minimal waist size.

To measure your trouser waist size, run your hand down your side and feel the top of your hip bone. Place a tape measure one inch above this on each side. It may help if you draw a line with a marker on your skin as a guide. Run the tape measure from your back around to your front, keeping it an inch above your hip bones on each side and the same distance from the floor all the way around. Before you measure, let out your breath and pull the tape snug against your skin but not so tight that it makes an indentation.

The average waist size of a representative group of adult American women measured in this way is thirty-seven inches and ranges from twenty-two to seventy inches. For women who still have menstrual periods, the average is an inch smaller, while for women who do not, it is about two inches larger. The table below shows the average percentage of fat for women with different waist sizes. If your waist size is larger than fifty inches, add 1 percent for each additional inch.

Estimating Your Percentage of Body Fat from Your Waist Size

Waist, in Inches	Percentage of Body Fat
22	24
23	25
24	28
25	29
26	30
27	31
28	33
29	34
30	35
31	36
32	39
33	40
34	41
35	42
36	43
37	43
38	44
39	45
40	45
41	45
42	46
43	47
44	47
45	48
46	48
47	49

48	49
49	50
50	50
51	51
52	52
53	53
54	55

Unlike their BMIs, Laurie's and Melanie's waist sizes do reflect the difference in their percentage of body fat. Laurie's waist size is twenty-five inches, while Melanie's is thirty-two inches, seven inches larger. If we look at the table, we will see that Laurie's waist indicates 29 percent fat while Melanie's matches to 39 percent, the same as their fat percentages on the electronic scale. So by using both BMI and waist size, you can get a better idea of your percentage of fat. If the percentage estimated from your waist size is higher than the average for your BMI, you have a larger-than-average waist size and so more fat; if it is smaller, then your waist size is smaller than average, which is healthier.

As we can see from all of their measurements, Laurie has fifteen pounds more muscle than Melanie and fifteen pounds less fat, but because the two happen to cancel each other out, they have the same overall weight. In addition to having more muscle than average, Laurie has a lower percentage of fat than would be expected for her BMI. If Laurie had the same amount of fat as Melanie, she would weigh fifteen pounds more. So muscle and fat both make their own contribution to weight, and this is why it is useful to estimate both.

There are several other better methods that can also be used to estimate your percentage of body fat. Electronic scales, like the one Laurie and Melanie used, estimate your fat percentage by measuring how well your skin conducts electricity (bioelectrical impedance). Because fat does not conduct electricity as well as more watery tissues, the more fat there is under your skin, the more electrical current is required to overcome its resistance. This method is not very accurate—it tends to underestimate your percentage of fat—but it's simple and inexpensive.

Weighing your body under water (hydrostatic weighing) or using a special X-ray machine (dual-energy X-ray absorptiometry) gives more accurate estimates, but these are more costly. The values for body fat for American women given in this book are based on the X-ray method. The most accurate method of all requires injecting radioactive material into the blood, but the X-ray method seems fairly comparable to this. Even if you have had your percentage of body fat measured by one of these methods, it may still be useful for you to estimate your percentage of fat from your BMI and waist size.

Putting It All Together

Now that you have seen how you can estimate your natural weight and BMI, body type, and body fat, we can put this information together. Let's take a look at the mother-daughter example we've used previously in the book, Susan and Jessica, to show what their approximate natural weights would be.

Measurements	Susan	Jessica
Age	45	22
Height (inches)	64	64
Weight (pounds)	166	146
BMI	28	25
Elbow (centimeters)	5.8	5.8
Wrist (centimeters)	4.9	4.9
Shoulder width (inches)	14	14
Hip width (inches)	11	11
Waist size (inches)	36	32
Current Estimates		
Percentage of fat, from BMI	43	38
Percentage of fat, from waist	43	39
Pounds of fat, from BMI	69	59

Estimated Natural Values	Susan	Jessica
Natural weight, from family	145	120
Natural weight, from graph	145	125
Adjusted for muscle	145	125
Natural BMI, from table	25	21

In the table above you can see all the measurements and estimates for Susan and Jessica. When they estimate their natural weights from the weights of their older female relatives, Susan looks back to her mother Helen at age forty-five and comes up with an estimate of 145 pounds; Jessica bases her estimate on her mother Susan's youthful weight of 120. Next, they each find where they fall along the line of today's women's weights and see what the corresponding natural weight would be. For Susan, her present weight of 166 corresponds to a natural weight of 145; Jessica's current weight of 145 lines up with a natural weight of 125. So these two estimation methods agree perfectly for Susan and differ by only five pounds for Jessica.

Because their bone measurements are average for their height, they do not need to adjust this estimate to account for having more or less muscle. This means that they both have average body types. If their bone measurements were higher than average, they would add some weight to their estimates, like Laurie, and if they were lower than average, they would subtract some pounds, like Melanie. Susan's and Jessica's percentages of fat estimated from their BMI and waist sizes also agree, which shows that their waist sizes are average for their heights and weights.

Susan's and Jessica's estimated natural weights show that if they can return to the same kind of diet that Susan's mother had for most of her life, their natural weights should each be about twenty pounds lower than their current weights. And because their natural BMIs would also be much lower, Jessica would be at the lower end of the normal range instead of being overweight, and Susan would be at the low end of the overweight range instead of the high end, where she is now.

As a reminder, your estimated natural weight is not a goal; nor is it a number you can achieve by a restricted-calorie weight-loss diet. You might get down to this weight with such a diet, but your lost pounds will almost certainly come right back, just as they have in the past for both Susan and Jessica. Rather, by permanently changing to a more natural diet and following the guidelines we have given in the previous chapters, women like Susan and Jessica will find that their weights will *gradually* go down over a period of many months, just as they did for Valerie Frankel. It took many years for women like Susan and Jessica to accumulate their excess weight, so it will also take some time to shed it.

That is why it is very important for you to find a mix of more natural foods that you will find appealing and satisfying over the long haul and stick with it. It does not have to be like anyone else's dietary pattern, as long as you like it and it conforms to our basic guidelines. There are many different food choices that conform to a natural diet and to our guidelines. Virtually all the choices that a woman would have had forty years ago or that European women still have, with much less omega-6 and much more omega-3, should be fine. With a sustainable natural diet that you enjoy, you should have the sustained pleasure of seeing your body shape and weight gradually move back to where they should have been. To help to inspire you, you can make similar tables for yourself by putting in your measurements and the average values from the tables on the indicated pages on the blank worksheet below.

Your Body Measurements

Measurements						
Age						
Height (inches)						
Weight (pounds)						
BMI (weight x 720)÷(height x height)						
Elbow (centimeters)						

Wrist (centimeters)						
Shoulder width (inches)						
Hip width (inches)						
Waist size (inches)						

Your Bone Measurements

If your measurement is higher or lower than the average, multiply the difference by the weight adjustment factor and that will be the change in pounds.

	Measurements			Averages (from Table on Page 186)	Weight Adjustment	Change in Pounds	
Elbow					1 mm = 5 lbs.		
Wrist					1 mm = 5 lbs.		
Shoulder					1 inch = 24 lbs.		
Hips					1 inch = 20 lbs.		
				Sum			
				Divide sum by 4 for average			

Your Current and Natural Body Type

Current Estimates	Reference Table (Page)		
Weight adjustment factor	187		
Percentage of fat, from BMI	189		
Percentage of fat, from waist	191		
Pounds of fat, from BMI	189		
Estimated natural values			
Natural weight, from family			
Natural weight, from graph	179–80		
Adjusted for muscle			
Natural BMI, from table	181		

It's Not Your Fault If You're Heavy, but You Don't Have to Be This Heavy

On an early fall day in 2008, an archaeology student who was part of a team from the University of Tübingen was sifting through the clay at the bottom of a nine-foot-deep hole inside the Hohle Fels cave in southwestern Germany when she found a small piece of carved ivory. The layer of clay she was working in had been deposited there about forty thousand years ago. The next day the team found a larger piece of ivory in the trench, and when the archaeologist in charge of the dig, Nicholas Conard, brushed off the dirt, he was very delighted to see that it was the carved figure of a woman. Over the next few days, the team found four more ivory fragments. Pieced together, they reveal the "Venus of Hohle Fels," an intricately carved two-and-a-half-inch figure of a woman with large breasts, hips, and thighs, and looking like she might be pregnant. At the top is a carved ring so that it could be worn as a pendant. The dating of this sculpture to around forty thousand years ago makes it the oldest example of figurative art ever found.

But this is just one of more than two hundred similar Stone Age "Venus figurines" that have been found spread out over distances of more than three thousand miles, from southern Spain to Russia. While a few reveal slender figures with low waist–hip ratios, most depict women with an abundance of fat even by current American standards. There is no way to know just why Stone Age people made so many of these figures and how and why they were spread out over such a vast distance. But it seems likely that they recognized that there is a connection between women's fat and her ability to have children. Our ancient ancestors seem to have believed that having fat was very valuable for women. But today, we seem to have lost this ancient insight.

The stories in Gina Kolata's reports on the weekly sessions of a group of obese men and women participating in a weight-loss program are quite sad. Even though their previous attempts to lose weight and *keep it off* had failed, the group's members all believed that this time would be different. And when the pounds were coming off, as they usually do at first, they were even more certain that this time they would succeed, and they were full of hope, pride, and self-assurance. Then, as it almost always does, the lost weight came back. All of their cheerful optimism, pride, and pleasure at losing weight gradually turned to bitter feelings of failure and regret. But this is not an isolated event involving a few unfortunate souls; millions of American women have this same experience every year. We do the same thing again and again, each time expecting the result to be different from what it was before. It's very difficult for us to accept that there may be built-in biological limits that shape what we weigh even when we experience these limits over and over again.

We know from studies of twins that your weight in your late teens is mostly shaped by your genes and your time in the womb. And we have seen how gaining weight after childbirth is also programmed into a woman's genes so that she can have bigger, healthier children. Because adding fat benefits her children, her genes are determined to make this happen. So for better or worse, our weight destinies are determined very early in our lives, and there are strict limits to how much we can alter them. Once we are again eating a normal and natural diet by getting our omega-6s and omega-3s back in balance and our weight has fallen to its natural level, we may be able to control another five or ten pounds at best.

But Americans find it very difficult to accept limits; it is one of the main things that has made our country great. We believe passionately that our lives are in our own hands and that we are not limited in any fundamental way in what we can accomplish. Whatever our circumstances, we are still free to find our own destiny, and no one should tell us that we can't. Because of our conviction that we are free to live in any way we choose and achieve whatever goals we set for ourselves, we find it difficult to accept that there may be some limits that are difficult to transcend. Our whole national identity is based on the belief that no matter what circumstances you are born in, you can accomplish almost anything if you are willing to work hard and give it your all. So it is natural for us to believe that how much we weigh is within our control and subject to our will and that we can control it if we just try hard enough, and it is not surprising that most American women share that belief.

But the belief that we can escape our biological limits can have unfortunate consequences. More than forty years ago, an eight-month-old baby boy named David was the innocent victim of a botched circumcision. His parents consulted with a highly regarded academic psychologist who strongly believed that our minds are not shaped by our biology, but only by our experience. He recommended that they have David's testicles removed and raise him as a girl. This was done, and he was given the name Brenda. At first this seemed to be working, and "Brenda's" story was written up as a stunning example of how our sexual identity is learned rather than being inborn. But it wasn't true; "Brenda" was still behaving like a boy even after he was given estrogen hormone; and the older he grew, the more unhappy and frustrated he became. Finally, when he was thirteen, his parents finally told him the truth, and he immediately took steps to become the boy he had always felt himself to be. David's full and rather tragic story was only told years later in the book *As Nature Made Him: The Boy Who Was Raised as a Girl.*

There certainly are biological and genetic programs that we can transcend by using our wits and our will, but what sex we are is not one of them. Our destined weight is not as fixed as our sex, but it is still mostly set when we are born. A woman's weight at the end of her childhood and how much she gains after having children are largely determined by her genes and by her own experience in her mother's womb.

Because a variety of different genes determines your weight and because these genes are constantly shuffled and mixed during the formation of egg and sperm cells, some women will happen to have a mix of genes that makes them naturally quite thin, some will have a combination that makes them quite heavy, and most will be spread out in between. It is possible for a naturally heavy woman to be thin only if she is willing to live in a state of perpetual semistarvation and constant exercise. Even those who undergo surgical procedures to bypass or limit the size of their stomachs will usually begin regaining weight over time. At the same time, some naturally thin women can tuck away enormous numbers of calories without gaining an ounce, just like Ethan Sim's student volunteers, much to the dismay of their heavier friends. It all depends on how your particular deck of gene-cards happens to be shuffled and the luck of your draw.

But while the influence of our genes is undeniable, the increased weight gain that American women have been experiencing over the past fifty years is not part of our biological destiny. Instead, it seems to be the result of our adopting a diet very different from any that humans have ever had before. We made these changes partly because we were told that this would make us healthier even though there was no evidence that they would and no evidence that they did. The enormous increase of purified vegetable oils high in omega-6 fats in our diets and the loss of much of our omega-3 is not necessary or biologically ordained. We can choose to give up this diet and return to one that doesn't cause this kind of excessive weight gain, like the diet that we used to have in the middle of the twentieth century and which millions of Europeans still have. If we are willing to do this, there is a good chance that our weights will gradually return to a more normal level. Though much of our weight is predetermined—especially at the time of life when women bear children—the good news is there *is* something that we can do about the weight that troubles us the most. That part of our destiny is still in our own hands.

APPENDIX

Fats

Major Fat Types	Saturated	Monounsaturated	Polyunsaturated	
First double bond	none	omega-9	omega-6	omega-3
Simple forms	many	oleic	linoleic	alpha-linolenic
Active forms	many	oleic	arachidonic	EPA, DHA
Common dietary sources	animal fat, meat, dairy	olive oil, canola oil	corn, corn oil, soybean oil, cornfed meat	fish, and other seafood, flaxseed oil, canola oil
Major effects	dairy healthy	lower weight, better health	increased weight and inflammation	lower weight and inflammation

Foods High in Omega-6 Linoleic Acid to Avoid

This table is based on the current USDA Nutrient Database, but values are subject to change.

Food Groups	Percentage of Linoleic
Meat, Eggs, and Dairy	
Flauta with chicken	19
Moo shu pork with pancake	12

Bacon bits, meat substitute	12
Fatback, salt pork	10
Fried chicken chunks, nuggets, wings (coated)	8
Breakfast sausage link, patty, meat substitute	8
Turkey bacon	7
Chicken salad spread	6
Soft shell crab (breaded)	6
Scrambled eggs from mix (cholesterol free or with cheese)	6
Fried chicken drumsticks, thighs, legs	5–6
Fish sandwich, crab salad, fried chicken fillet	6
Kung pao, lemon, or General Tso chicken (prepared)	5–6
Tuna, chicken, turkey, ham, pork, salmon salad (prepared)	5–6
Fish sticks, fish floured or breaded	5
Samosa pastry with potatoes and peas, tamales	5
Pasta with pesto sauce, chimichanga, taquitos, fritters	5
Macaroni or pasta salad with egg, crab, tuna	4–5
Hamburger with mayo, tomato, and bun	4
Chicken or turkey cake, patty, croquette	4
Floured or breaded fish, shrimp, scallops	4
Pork chop (breaded and fried)	4
Pork rinds (deep-fried)	4
Pork, turkey, or Polish sausage, hot dog, bologna	4
Eggs, cheese, sausage or bacon on biscuit or muffin	4
Meat substitute, sandwich spread, chicken	4
Luncheon meats, sausage	3–4
Beef steak (breaded, floured, battered, baked, or fried)	3
Pizza (thin or thick crust), pizza with meat, egg rolls	3
Quiche, calzone, quesadilla with meat	3
Vegetables and Fruits	
White potato chips, potato sticks	20

White potato chips (reduced fat)	11
Pea salad, cabbage salad, or coleslaw	8–10
Mustard sauce	10
Chocolate topping (Smucker's magic shell)	9
French fries, hash browns	7
Onion rings	7
Fried green tomatoes	6
Vegetables with batter or cooked with fat	5
Salsa (red)	4
Chiles rellenos, stuffed mushrooms, cucumber salad	3
Eggplant parmesan, vegetable tempura	3
Baked Goods and Cereals	
Popcorn (popped in oil)	22
Puff pastry	20
Salty snacks, corn puffs, corn chips, pretzels	14–16
Granola bars	8–12
Chocolate fudge cookie bars	12
Carrot cake, zucchini cake	10
Cookies (sugar wafer, almond, chocolate chip)	8
Sweet rolls, coffee cake, cinnamon buns	8
Crackers (including whole wheat)	8
Salty snacks (e.g., corn puffs)	8
Muffins (with fruit, nuts, zucchini, wheat bran), corn bread	7–8
Dietetic cookie, sandwich, chocolate chip	7
Vanilla cookies (French cream, Cameo, Chalet)	7
Hush puppies, biscuits	6
Wheat germ cereal	6
Cereal (Banana Nut Crunch cereal, Reese's Puffs, oat bran)	5
Bread sticks, garlic bread	5
Fruit pastries, pound cake, apple pie, cookies, brownies	5

Pies, biscotti, churros, lemon cake, Danish, fruit bars	4
Taco shells	4
Whole-wheat bread, cracked-wheat bread, cheese roll	3
Nuts, Seeds, Oils, and Dressings	
Sunflower seed oil	65
Corn oil	53
Cottonseed oil	52
Soybean oil	52
"Vegetable oil"	43
Mayonnaise dressing	41
Peppercorn dressing	38
Liquid margarine	33
Caesar dressing	29
Tartar sauce	25
Blue cheese or Roquefort or sesame dressing	24
Margarine-like spreads	24
Solid margarine	23
Creamy dressing	22
Fruit dressing with honey, oil, water	18
French dressing	18
Thousand Island dressing	16
Italian dressing (oil and vinegar)	13
Nut rolls, Reese's Peanut Butter Cups	5–6

Foods High in Omega-3 to Add to the Diet

This table is based primarily on the current USDA Nutrient Database.

Foods High in DHA and EPA	**Percentage of DHA***
Fish oil	11–33
Fish (see the "Fish," table on page 207)	0.1–1.8

Omega-3-enriched eggs	0.4
Oysters	0.3
Crab	0.2
Shrimp	0.1
Clams	0.1
Grass-fed chicken	0.1
Game animals (deer, elk)	0.05
Lobster	0.03
Grass-fed beef or bison	0.02
Foods High in Alpha-Linolenic	*Percentage of Alpha-Linolenic*
Flaxseed oil	53
Flaxseeds	23
Walnut oil	10
Canola oil	9
Walnuts	9

* Percentages of EPA are usually similar to DHA.

Fish and Seafood

Percentage of DHA and EPA in fish and seafood, and mercury content where available.

Fish or Seafood	DHA percentage	EPA percentage	Mercury (parts per million)
roe	1.75	1.26	can be high
salmon, Atlantic	1.45	0.69	0.014
shad	1.31	1.09	0.044
anchovy	1.29	0.76	0.043
whitefish	1.21	0.41	0.069
mackerel, Pacific	1.20	0.65	0.088
tuna, bluefin, fresh	1.14	0.36	0.118
herring	1.11	0.91	0.044
mackerel, Spanish	0.95	0.29	**0.2–0.5**

salmon, coho	0.87	0.41	0.014
salmon, canned	0.82	0.77	very low
tilefish	0.73	0.17	**1.45**
salmon, cooked	0.71	0.51	0.014
mackerel, Atlantic	0.70	0.50	0.050
white tuna in water	0.69	0.23	**0.430**†
trout	0.68	0.26	0.072
swordfish	0.68	0.14	**0.976**
bluefish	0.67	0.32	**0.337**
sea bass	0.56	0.21	0.219
shark	0.53	0.32	**0.998**
sardines, canned	0.51	0.47	0.016
bass, freshwater	0.46	0.31	can be high
pollock	0.45	0.09	0.041
halibut	0.37	0.09	0.252
oysters	0.30	0.88	0.013
snapper	0.27	0.05	0.189
whiting	0.24	0.28	very low
blue crab	0.23	0.24	0.060
king mackerel	0.23	0.17	**0.730**
perch	0.22	0.10	0.014
light tuna in water	0.22	0.05	0.078†
tuna, albacore	0.22	0.05	**0.353**†
grouper	0.21	0.04	**0.465**
haddock	0.16	0.08	0.031
cod	0.15	0.09	0.095
mullet	0.15	0.18	0.046
carp	0.15	0.31	0.140
clams	0.15	0.14	very low
shrimp	0.14	0.17	very low

catfish*	0.13	0.05	0.049
tilapia*	0.13	0.01	low
king crab	0.12	0.30	0.060
flounder; sole	0.11	0.10	0.045
scallops	0.10	0.09	0.050
croaker	0.10	0.12	0.072
orange roughy	0.08	0.21	**0.554**
crayfish	0.04	0.12	0.033
pike	0.03	0.07	**high**
lobster, northern	0.03	0.05	**0.310**
sushi	0.01	0.03	**can be high**

EPA and DHA percentages are from the USDA Nutrient Database. Higher mercury levels are marked in bold. Some items have not been tested.

* These fish have high levels of omega-6 when farmed.

† Some canned tuna may have higher amounts; see Consumer Reports, January 2011; most mercury levels from www.health.gov/dietaryguidelines/dga2005/report/html/table_g2_adda2.htm; and www.fda.gov /food/foodsafety/product-specificinformation/seafood/foodbornepathogenscontaminants/methylmercury /ucm115644.htm.

Better Fast Foods (Less than 1 percent Linoleic)

(MD = McDonald's, BK = Burger King, TB = Taco Bell, JB = Jack-in-the-Box, DQ = Dairy Queen)

Note: These values are based on the USDA Nutrient Database and are subject to change. Check the nutrition and ingredient information at the restaurant.

Item	Percentage of Linoleic
Dairy	
milk, yogurt	0.1
fruit and yogurt parfait (MD)	0.1
carry-out milk shake (MD, BK, DQ, Carl's Jr., Roy Rogers)	0.1
frozen yogurt	0.2
cheese, cheese nuggets	0.2
soft serve ice cream (MD, DQ)	0.3

Meats	
shrimp, steamed or boiled, no batter	0.1
sushi	0.1
chicken and rice soup	0.2
chicken or turkey Caesar garden salad (MD, Wendy's)	0.3
beef, broiled or baked	0.4
chicken, not fried or coated, no skin	0.4
meat loaf with beef	0.4
pastrami sandwich	0.5
chicken teriyaki	0.5
chili	0.5
turkey, ham, and roast beef club sandwich, with lettuce, tomato (Subway)	0.6
beef and potatoes	0.7
chicken submarine sandwich, with lettuce, tomato (Subway, Jerry's)	0.7
soft taco with beef, cheese, lettuce, tomato, salsa/sour cream (TB)	0.7
burrito with beef or chicken, beans, cheese, or rice, sour cream (TB)	0.7–0.8
croissant sandwich, ham and cheese (Arby's)	0.8
sweet and sour pork or chicken	0.8
taco or tostada with beef, beans, cheese, flower tortilla (TB)	0.8
roast beef sandwich with cheese (Arby's, JB)	0.8
double cheese burger, with tomato and/or ketchup (MD)	0.9
roast beef sandwich (Arby's, Hardee's, Roy Rogers)	0.9
Baked Goods, Pasta, Grains	
rice, grits	0.1
pasta with tomato sauce, cheese	0.2
tortellini, cheese, tomato sauce	0.3
wonton soup	0.4
steamed dumplings with meat or seafood	0.4

ravioli, with tomato sauce	0.6
bread: rye, French, sourdough, Cuban	0.7
roll, sourdough	0.7
Italian pie (meatless) (Pizza Hut)	0.7
pancakes, sourdough	0.8
croissants	0.8
Vegetables and Fruits	
candy, no icing	0.0
lettuce salad with tomatoes, carrots, no dressing	0.05
potato, baked or mashed	0.1
shrimp garden salad, no dressing (MD)	0.1
salsa (but not chips or de chile rojo)	0.1
salad greens	0.1
fruit juice, salad, fruit	0.1
shrimp garden salad, no dressing (MD)	0.1
fruit and yogurt parfait (MD)	0.1
chicken or turkey garden salad, no dressing	0.2
julienne salad, meat, cheese, eggs, vegetables, no dressing (BK, Hardee's, MD)	0.4
onion soup	0.5

Less Desirable Fast Foods and Condiments

(MD = McDonald's, BK = Burger King, JB = Jack-in-the-Box)

Note: These values are based on the USDA Nutrient Database and are subject to change.

Item	Percentage of Linoleic
mayonnaise	40
margarine	33
tartar sauce	24
Caesar dressing	29
creamy dressing	22
French dressing	18

salty snacks, corn puffs	17
Thousand Island dressing	16
chow mein	15
Italian dressing	12
potato chips	12
moo shu pork	12
bacon bits, meatless	12
potato chips with reduced fat	11
egg salad	11
tortilla chips	9
chocolate chip cookie	8
butterscotch or brownie cookie	7
chicken patty, tenders, or fillet, breaded (BK, KFC)	7
chicken or turkey salad	7
sweet roll	7
french fries	7
onion rings	7
nachos with cheese	6
biscuits (MD, Hardee's, Popeyes, KFC)	6
chicken fillet (breaded and fried) sandwich (Wendy's, Carl's Jr., JB, MD, BK)	6
coleslaw	6
fried fish sandwich	6
kung pao chicken	6
fried chicken fillet	6
double cheeseburger, mayo or salad dressing, double bun (MD)	5
bread stick	5
chicken nuggets	5
chicken wings	5
hash brown potatoes (MD, Hardee's, Carl's Jr., JB)	5

tuna salad	5
chicken salad sandwich	5
fried apple pie (MD)	5
salty snacks, multigrain	5
bread stick, garlic bread	4-5
egg, cheese, and sausage or bacon on biscuit	4
brownie	4
Danish	3
potato salad	3

AUTHORS' NOTE

Much of the information presented in this book is from our original research. This research is based on our own analysis of data from a variety of sources. Most of our findings relating to American women come from our analysis of raw data from the U.S. National Health and Nutrition Examination Surveys (NHANES) done in 1971–75, 1976–80, 1988–94, 1999–2000, 2001–2, 2003–4, 2005–6, and 2007–8. This includes data for height, weight, BMI, body fat, waist and hip sizes and ratios, detailed diet records, exercise patterns, blood pressure, and blood chemistries. Figures for bone, fat, and nonfat amounts and percentages in American women are based on dual-energy X-ray absorptiometry values from the NHANES 2003–4. Data for average shoulder, hip, elbow, and wrist widths, and hip circumference are from the NHANES III 1988–94. Data on heights and weights were also used from the National Health Examination Surveys of 1959–62 and 1963–65. Data relating to women's lowest weights after age eighteen comes from the NHANES I 1971–75 and NHANES 1999–2000. The raw data sets for all of these surveys are available at www.cdc.gov/nchs /nhanes/nhanes_questionnaires.htm.

When we use the term "average," that refers to the average, or mean, value. When we use the term "typical" for a value, that refers to the median value, the value in the middle of all values, which may be more representative. When we give weights that correspond to BMIs, we use the weight of an American woman of average height, sixty-four inches. Weights tend to change by about five pounds when height changes by one inch. When we say "now" or "today," we are usually referring to the NHANES for 2007–8, though in some cases it will be the 2003–4 or 2004–5 surveys for data items not yet available for the later survey. In fact, just before this book went to the printer, special data on fatty acids in the blood plasma of 951 American women twenty and older was released as a supplement to the NHANES survey 2003–4. The data includes about a third of the women in that survey group. Though that is a relatively small number, analysis of the new data strongly supports the ideas expressed in this book. As in other studies, the amount of omega-3 DHA in American women's blood is strongly linked to lower weights, while omega-6 arachidonic is strongly linked to higher weights. This effect is especially strong in women under sixty years of age.

Of the four types of omega-3, the amount of DHA in the blood is the form of omega-3 most strongly related to lower weights. Women with high levels of DHA in their blood weigh about forty pounds less than the women with low levels. Further supporting our argument, the women in this group with high levels of arachidonic (omega-6) weigh about forty pounds more than women with lower levels. Just as we found in the studies discussed earlier in the book, women in this study with higher DHA and lower arachidonic have the lowest weights.

This new blood fatty acid data also allows us to compare American women with women in Japan, a group with very low obesity rates and a diet high in omega-3 and low in omega-6. The Japanese women have more than *three times* as much omega-3 DHA in their blood as American women, while the Americans have one and a half times more omega-6 arachidonic. Those American women with blood DHA levels similar to the Japanese women have a BMI of 23 compared with 29 for the average American woman in this sample and just a little higher than the average BMI of 22 for Japanese women. This corresponds to a difference of about thirty pounds in weight. (For the Japanese studies, search for 21099130 and 15298193 at www.ncbi.nlm.nih.gov/pubmed.)

Also, as we would expect, women with more gamma-tocopherol in their blood from soybean and corn oil have higher levels of omega-6 arachidonic and lower levels of omega-3 DHA in their blood. Those with high levels of gamma-tocopherol have one-third less DHA than those with low levels. This supports the idea that having more omega-6 fat in the diet reduces the amount of DHA in the blood. Also as expected, women with more arachidonic tend to have higher amounts of fat in the belly, while those with more DHA tend to have more fat in their legs. Finally, women have higher levels of DHA than men, and the more children a woman has, the lower her DHA tends to be, as found in other studies. So, like the rest of the NHANES findings, these brand-new data strongly support many of the key ideas in this book. We very much appreciate the sacrifices of those who agreed to participate in these surveys.

Figures on changes in the American diet over time are based on several data sources compiled by the U.S. Department of Agriculture. Data on loss-adjusted food availability are available at www.ers.usda .gov/Data/foodconsumption/FoodGuideSpreadsheets.htm#calories. Data on nutrients in the American food supply are available at www .ers.usda.gov/Data/FoodConsumption/NutrientAvailIndex.htm and in the *Nutrient Content of the U.S. Food Supply* publications for 1909–97 and 2005.

Data on the fatty acid and nutrient composition of different foods in the American diet are from the USDA National Nutrient Database for Standard Reference. We have used the values of omega-3 and omega-6 in foods given in this database and in the diet records of American women in recommending which foods are good or bad to eat, but food compositions can change and some changes may not be reflected in the USDA's analyses. Unfortunately, there is no good alternative, since food makers are not obligated to provide information about the fatty acid content of their foods. The USDA database is available in a detailed format at www.nal.usda.gov/fnic/foodcomp/ search/ and in an easier-to-use format at http://199.133.10.140/code searchwebapp/(dcmyzbutway2pej42rukc055)/codesearch.aspx.

The data on the per capita food supply in the United States and other countries we have used come from the Food Balance Sheets of the United Nations Food and Agricultural Organization which include data for 117 food categories for 169 countries from 1961 to 2007 and are available at http://faostat.fao.org/site/368/DesktopDefault.aspx ?PageID=368#ancor.

We have estimated the amounts of omega-6 and omega-3 fats for each country at different times based on the foods included in the Food Balance Sheets and the composition of those foods in the USDA National Nutrient Database. Since the same food may differ in its composition in different countries and at different times, this may make these estimates less accurate. We have assumed that American soybean oil is either partially hydrogenated or the low-omega-3 type. Data on the composition of maternal milk in different countries comes from our compilation of values from more than two hundred published reports and from the analysis of Tsimane milk by our colleagues listed in the acknowledgments.

Figures on the average BMI and overweight and obesity rates in women in 195 countries in 2005 are from the World Health Organization Global Database on Body Mass Index at www.who.int/bmi. Weights for women in other countries are based on the average BMI and a height of sixty-four inches, the average for American women. Figures on infant and child mortality and age-adjusted mortality rates for different causes of death are from World Health Organization data available at www.who.int/healthinfo/statistics/mortality/en/index.html. Analyses of the relationships between diet, BMI, and mortality in different countries use data from all of these UN sources. Data on U.S. mortality rates and life expectancy come from the National Center for Health Statistics and are available at www.cdc.gov/nchs/deaths.htm. Data on per capita cigarette consumption from 1900 to 2007 in the United States come from the Tobacco Outlook Report, Economic

Research Service, U.S. Department of Agriculture. These are available at www.infoplease.com/ipa/A0908700.html.

Our analyses in chapter 4 of the risks of obstructed labor and Caesarian section in women with different parities and the relationships between parity, birth weight, and infant mortality are based on our analysis of data from the 1990 Birth Cohort Linked Birth/Infant Death Data Set (CD-ROM Series 20, No. 6). For the risks of obstructed labor, C-sections, and preeclampsia in women with different prepregnancy weights, we used data from the National Maternal and Infant Health Survey of 1988: www.cdc.gov/nchs/nvss/nmihs.htm. Recent figures about American births, including risks of preeclampsia and eclampsia, are based on tabulations of natality data available at http://205.207.175.93/vitalstats/ReportFolders/ReportFolders.aspx?IF _ActivePathName=P/Births/DataFiles.

NOTES

xii **low weights have been typical:** The average weight of women in their late teens in sixty-eight countries is based on data from Phyllis B. Eveleth and James M. Tanner's *Worldwide Variation in Human Growth*, 2nd ed. (New York: Cambridge University Press, 1990).

xiii **1890s, until the 1970s:** For average weights in American women over time, see Amanda M. Czerniawski, "From Average to Ideal: The Evolution of the Height and Weight Table in the United States, 1836–1943," *Social Science History* 31 (2007): 273–96.

xv **memory game:** See Donald H. McBurney, Steven J. C. Gaulin, Trishul Deviveni, and Christine Adams, "Superior Spatial Memory of Women: Stronger Evidence for the Gathering Hypothesis," *Evolution and Human Behavior* 18 (1997): 165–74.

xv **farmers' market:** See Joshua New, Max M. Krasnow, Danielle Truxaw, and Steven J. C. Gaulin, "Spatial Adaptations for Plant Foraging: Women Excel and Calories Count," *Proceedings of the Royal Society B* 274 (2007): 2679–84.

3 **Chapter 1:** The figures about American women in this chapter are based mainly on NHANES data for 2005–8. Mortality data are from the World Health Organization. Figures relating to diet in the United States and other countries are from Food Balance Sheets from the UN Food and Agricultural Organization and from the USDA.

4 *no* **credible studies:** For more on the amazing history of the diet-heart theory and the astonishing lack of evidence to support it see Gary Taubes, *Good Calories, Bad Calories: Challenging the Conventional Wisdom on Diet,*

Weight Control, and Disease (New York: Alfred A. Knopf, 2007); A. H. Hite, R. D. Feinman, G. E. Guzman, M. Satin, P. A. Schoenfeld, and R. J. Wood, "In the Face of Contradictory Evidence: Report of the Dietary Guidelines for Americans Committee," *Nutrition* 26 (2010): 915–24; George V. Mann, "Diet-Heart: End of an Era," *New England Journal of Medicine* 297 (1977): 644–50; E. H. Ahrens, Jr., "Diet and Heart Disease: Shaping Public Perceptions When Proof Is Lacking," *Arteriosclerosis* 2 (1982): 85–86; Uffe Ravnskov, Christian Allen, Dale Atrens, Mary G. Enig, Barry Groves, et al., "Studies of Dietary Fat and Heart Disease," *Science* 295 (2002): 1464–66; R. H. Rosenman, "The Independent Roles of Diet and Serum Lipids in the 20th-Century Rise and Decline of Coronary Heart Disease Mortality," *Integrative Physiological & Behavioral Science* 28 (1993): 84–98; William G. Rothstein, "Dietary Fat, Coronary Heart Disease, and Cancer: A Historical Review," *Preventive Medicine* 43 (2006): 356–60; William G. Rothstein, *Public Health and the Risk Factors: A History of an Uneven Medical Revolution* (Rochester, N.Y.: University of Rochester Press, 2003); Lars Werko, "End of the Road for the Diet-Heart Theory?" *Scandinavian Cardiovascular Journal* 42 (2008): 250–55; Thomas J. Moore, *Heart Failure: A Critical Inquiry into American Medicine and the Revolution in Heart Care* (New York: Random House, 1989); Sylvan Lee Weinberg, "The Diet-Heart Hypothesis: A Critique," *Journal of the American College of Cardiology* 43 (2004): 731–33.

4 **forty-eight thousand middle-aged American women:** Barbara V. Howard, Linda Van Horn, Judith Hsia, JoAnn E. Manson, Marcia L. Stefanick, Sylvia Wassertheil-Smoller, Lewis H. Kuller, et al. "Low-Fat Dietary Pattern and Risk of Cardiovascular Disease: The Women's Health Initiative Randomized Controlled Dietary Modification Trial," *Journal of the American Medical Association* 295 (2006): 655–66.

5 **famous Framingham Heart Study:** Tavia Gordon, "The Framingham Diet Study: Diet and the Regulation of Serum Cholesterol," vol. 24, *The Framingham Study*, 1968. George V. Mann, "Diet-Heart: End of an Era," *New England Journal of Medicine* 297 (1977): 644–50.

5 **many other studies:** See, for example, A. B. Nichols, C. Ravenscroft, D. E. Lamphiear, and L. D. Ostrander, Jr., "Daily Nutritional Intake and Serum Lipid Levels: The Tecumseh Study," *American Journal of Clinical Nutrition* 29 (1976): 1384–92. WHO European Collaborative Group, "Multifactorial Trial in the Prevention of Coronary Heart Disease: 3. Incidence and Mortality Results," *European Heart Journal* 4 (1983): 141–47; J. T. Salonen, P. Puska, and H. Mustaniemi, "Changes in Morbidity and Mortality During Comprehensive Community Programme to Control Cardiovascular Diseases during 1972–7 in North Karelia," *British Medical Journal* 2 (1979): 1178–83; G. Neil Thomas, Bernard M. Y. Cheung, Sai Yin Ho, Duncan J. Macfarlane, Han Bing Deng, Sarah M. McGhee, et al., "Overview of Dietary Influences on Atherosclerotic Vascular Disease:

Epidemiology and Prevention," *Cardiovascular & Hematological Disorders Drug Targets* 7 (2007): 87–97; J. M. Ordovas, "Diet-Heart Hypothesis: Will Diversity Bring Reconciliation?" *American Journal of Clinical Nutrition* 82 (2005): 919–20. Daan Kromhout, "Diet and Coronary Heart Disease in the Zutphen Study," in *Prevention of Coronary Heart Disease: Diet, Lifestyle, and Risk Factors in the Seven Countries Study*, edited by Daan Kromhout, Alessandro Menotti, and Henry Blackburn (Norwell, Mass.: Kluwer Academic Publishers, 2002), 72–84; L. E. Ramsay, W. W. Yeo, and P. R. Jackson, "Dietary Reduction of Serum Cholesterol Concentration: Time to Think Again," *British Medical Journal* 303 (1991): 953–57.

5 **recent review:** W. Siri-Tarino, Qi Sun, Frank B. Hu, and Ronald M. Krauss, "Meta-Analysis of Prospective Cohort Studies Evaluating the Association of Saturated Fat with Cardiovascular Disease," *American Journal of Clinical Nutrition* 91 (2010): 535–46. See also Marion G. Volk, "An Examination of the Evidence Supporting the Association of Dietary Cholesterol and Saturated Fats with Serum Cholesterol and Development of Coronary Heart Disease," *Alternative Medicine Review* 12 (2007): 228–45.

5 **astonishing lack of scientific evidence:** A. H. Hite, R. D. Feinman, G. E. Guzman, M. Satin, P. A. Schoenfeld, and R. J. Wood, "In the Face of Contradictory Evidence: Report of the Dietary Guidelines for Americans Committee," *Nutrition* 26 (2010): 915–24.

5 **Ike's Multibillion-Dollar Heart Attack:** See Clarence G. Lasby, *Eisenhower's Heart Attack* (Lawrence: University of Kansas Press, 1997).

6 **press conference three days later:** See "Transcript of Heart Specialist's News Conference," *New York Times*, September 27, 1955, 21.

7 **ways the Italian diet was different:** See Food Balance Sheets for 1961 from the UN Food and Agricultural Organization.

7 **"Mediterranean diet":** Ancel Keys, "Mediterranean Diet and Public Health: Personal Reflections," *American Journal of Clinical Nutrition* 61 (1995): 1321S–23S.

7 **cholesterol levels in their blood:** Ancel Keys, "Atherosclerosis: A Problem in Newer Public Health," *Journal of the Mount Sinai Hospital, New York* 20 (1953): 118–39.

7 **connection between their diets and their blood cholesterol:** Ancel Keys, Joseph T. Anderson, and Francisco Grande, "Serum Cholesterol in Man: Diet Fat and Instrinsic Responsiveness," *Circulation* 19 (1959): 201–14. The same thing was found in almost every population studied; see, for example, Daan Kromhout, Alessandro Menotti, and Henry Blackburn, editors, *Prevention of Coronary Heart Disease: Diet, Lifestyle, and Risk Factors in the Seven Countries Study* (Norwell, Mass.: Kluwer Academic Publishers, 2002).

8 **wrote up his wonderful new idea:** Ancel Keys, "Atherosclerosis: A Problem in Newer Public Health," *Journal of the Mount Sinai Hospital, New York* 20 (1953): 118–39, esp. 134.

8 **as other researchers soon pointed out:** J. Yerushalmy and Herman E. Hilleboe, "Fat in the Diet and Mortality from Heart Disease: A Methodologic Note," *New York State Journal of Medicine* 57 (1957): 2343–54.

8 **later critics:** See G. V. Mann, "Diet-Heart: End of an Era," *New England Journal of Medicine* 297 (1977): 644–50.

9 **deaths from heart disease in women:** Based on historical data from the U.S. National Vital Statistics System available at www.cdc.gov/nchs /nvss/mortality_historical_data.htm.

9 **cigarette smoking:** Based on data from the CDC at www.cdc.gov /tobacco/data_statistics/tables/economics/consumption/.

9 *Time* **magazine:** "Medicine: The Specialized Nubbin," *Time*, October 31, 1955.

9 *Reader's Digest*: Blake Clark, "Is This the No. 1 Villain in Heart Disease?" *Reader's Digest*, November 1955, 109–13.

9 **General Mills:** Victor J. Hillery, "Diet Fright," *Wall Street Journal*, August 14, 1957, 1.

9 **all but quoted Keys:** Advertisement in *Reader's Digest*, May 1957, 177.

10 **corn oil could actually lower cholesterol:** E. H. Ahrens, Jr., D. H. Blankenhorn, and T. T. Tsaltas, "Effect on Human Serum Lipids of Substituting Plant for Animal Fat in Diet," *Proceedings of the Society for Experimental Biology & Medicine* 86 (1954): 872–78; Carmel McCoubrey, "Edward Ahrens, Cholestrol Researcher, Is Dead at 85," *New York Times*, December 16, 2000.

10 **sitosterol:** R. E. Ostlund, Jr., S. B. Racette, A. Okeke, and W. F. Stenson, "Phytosterols That Are Naturally Present in Commercial Corn Oil Significantly Reduce Cholesterol Absorption in Humans," *American Journal of Clinical Nutrition* 75 (2002): 1000–1004.

10 **quickly confirmed this:** Ancel Keys, Joseph T. Anderson, and Francisco Grande, "Prediction of Serum-Cholesterol Responses of Man to Changes in Fats in the Diet," *Lancet* 273 (1957): 959–66.

10 **vice president modestly explained:** Quoted in Victor J. Hillery, "Diet Fright," *Wall Street Journal*, August 14, 1957, 1.

11 **Paul Dudley White, stunned his cohost:** Quoted in Mary Enig and Sally Fallon, "Oiling of America," *Nexus* 6/1–2 (1998–99).

11 **report poked holes:** Irvine H. Page, Frederick J. Stare, A. C. Corcoran, Herbert Pollack, and Charles F. Wilkinson, Jr., "Atherosclerosis and the Fat Content of the Diet," *Circulation* 16 (1957): 163–78. Robert K. Plumb, "Experts Disagree on Diet vs. Heart," *New York Times*, January 16, 1957, 33.

11 **not a very good predictor:** In the Framingham study of heart disease, for example, blood cholesterol was not related to heart disease in women nor in men over fifty. Thomas R. Dawber, *The Framingham Study: The Epidemiology of Atherosclerotic Disease* (Cambridge, Mass.: Harvard University Press, 1980).

11 **countries with fewer deaths:** See Ancel Keys, *Seven Countries* (Cambridge, Mass: Harvard University Press, 1980).

11 **diet-heart enthusiasts:** National Heart Lung and Blood Institute, "Consensus Conference: Lowering Blood Cholesterol to Prevent Heart Disease," *Journal of the American Medical Association* 253 (1985): 2080–86.

12 *Eat Well and Stay Well*: Ancel and Margaret Keys (New York: Doubleday, 1959).

12 **tried to stem this tide**: For FDA efforts see "Fat and Oil Ads Disputed by U.S.," *New York Times*, December 11, 1959, 26. Also: "Government Seizes Shredded Wheat Sold by National Biscuit Co.," *Wall Street Journal*, September 28, 1964, 8.

13 **endorse his views:** Irvine H. Page, Edgar V. Allen, Francis L. Chamberlain, Ancel Keys, Jeremiah Stamler, and Fredrick J. Stare, "Dietary Fat and Its Relation to Heart Attacks and Strokes," *Circulation* 23 (1961): 133–36.

13 *all* **Americans should reduce fat:** "Heart Association Stirs Up Controversy by Urging Public to Alter Intake of Fats," *Wall Street Journal*, June 10, 1964, 6.

13 **FDA found that most Americans:** "Oil-Food Labels Held Misleading," *New York Times*, May 28, 1964, 75.

13 *Dietary Goals* **put together:** U.S. Senate Select Committee on Nutrition and Human Needs, *Dietary Goals for the United States* (Washington, D.C.: U.S. Government Printing Office, 1977).

14 **no medical evidence to support the** *Dietary Goals*: Senate Select Committee on Nutrition and Human Needs, "Dietary Goals, Supplemental Views" (Washington, D.C.: U.S. Government Printing Office, 1977): statements by James Sammons, president of the American Medical Association, and Theodore Cooper, head of the National Heart and Lung Institute.

14 **Many other expert physicians:** See E. H. Ahrens, Jr., "Dietary Fats and Coronary Heart Disease: Unfinished Business," *Lancet* 2 (1979): 1345–48.

14 **George Mann:** Said Mann: "A large probability exists that the hydrogenated fats created during the industrial process are damaging to health because of their content of unnatural 'trans' isomers." Senate Select Committee on Nutrition and Human Needs, "Dietary Goals, Supplemental Views" (Washington, D.C.: U.S. Government Printing Office, 1977), 667.

14 **mollify the meat industry:** U.S. Senate Select Committee on Nutrition and Human Needs, *Dietary Goals for the United States*, 2nd ed. (Washington, D.C.: U.S. Government Printing Office, 1977). Senator Bob Dole asked to change the goal of reducing meat consumption to "decrease consumption of animal fat and choose meats, poultry and fish, which will reduce saturated fat intake."

14 **A 2010 review of the current** *Dietary Guidelines*: A. H. Hite, R. D. Feinman, G. E. Guzman, M. Satin, P. A. Schoenfeld, and R. J. Wood, "In the Face of Contradictory Evidence: Report of the Dietary Guidelines for Americans Committee," *Nutrition* 26 (2010): 915–24.

14 **most Americans believed:** "Oil-Food Labels Held Misleading," *New York Times*, May 28, 1964, 75; B. Schucker, K. Bailey, J. T. Heimbach, M. E. Mattson, J. T. Wittes, C. M. Haines, D. J. Gordon, J. A. Cutler, V. S. Keating, R. S. Goor, et al., "Change in Public Perspective on Cholesterol and Heart Disease: Results from Two National Surveys," *Journal of the American Medical Association* 258 (1987): 3527–31.

14–15 **most physicians still did not accept:** B. Schucker, J. T. Wittes, J. A. Cutler, K. Bailey, D. R. Mackintosh, D. J. Gordon, et al., "Change in Physician Perspective on Cholesterol and Heart Disease: Results from Two National Surveys," *Journal of the American Medical Association* 258 (1987): 3521–26.

15 **MRFIT study:** "Multiple Risk Factor Intervention Trial. Risk Factor Changes and Mortality Results. Multiple Risk Factor Intervention Trial Research Group," *Journal of the American Medical Association* 248 (1982): 1465–77.

15 **gave up on trying to show that changing the diet:** In 1971, a National Heart and Lung Institute task force recommended against funding a test of the diet-heart theory with one hundred thousand Americans and opted instead for the MRFIT study, which included diet along with smoking advice and blood pressure control and which failed to show any benefit.

15 **drugs were causing excessive numbers of deaths:** See Thomas J. Moore, *Heart Failure* (New York: Random House, 1989).

15 **finally found a drug:** See "The Lipid Research Clinics Coronary Primary Prevention Trial Results. I. Reduction in Incidence of Coronary Heart Disease," *Journal of the American Medical Association* 251 (1984): 351–64. For the lack of statistical significance in this study, see Richard A. Kronmal, "Commentary on the Published Results of the Lipid Research Clinics Coronary Primary Prevention Trial," *Journal of the American Medical Association* 253(14) (1985): 2091–93.

15 **"consensus conference":** See Thomas J. Moore, *Heart Failure* (New York: Random House, 1989). For the final report, see National Heart, Lung, and Blood Institute, "Consensus Conference. Lowering Blood Cholesterol to Prevent Heart Disease," *Journal of the American Medical Association* 253 (1985): 2080–86.

15 **testimony of a number of leading researchers:** Researchers testifying against the diet recommendation in the consensus report included Edward H. Ahrens, Jr., Eliot Corday, and Basil M. Rifkind.

15 **the panel went along with this:** The Advisory Committee for the National Heart, Lung, and Blood Institute, a separate group from the panel at the consensus conference, refused to approve funding for the new program, which was funded in another way. See Thomas Moore's *Heart Failure* for more details.

16 **no convincing evidence:** George V. Mann, "Diet-Heart: End of an Era," *New England Journal of Medicine* 297 (1977): 644–50.

16 **Keys himself later backed away:** Philip M. Boffey, "Cholesterol: Debate Flares over Wisdom in Widespread Reductions," *New York Times,* July 14, 1987, C1.

16 **Keys's own research:** A. Keys, A. Menotti, M. J. Karvonen, C. Aravanis, H. Blackburn, R. Buzina, B. S. Djordjevic, A. S. Dontas, F. Fidanza, and M. H. Keys, "The Diet and 15-Year Death Rate in the Seven Countries Study," *American Journal of Epidemiology* 124 (1986): 903–15.

17 **Chapter 2:** Original research in this chapter is based on food data from the UN Food and Agricultural Organization and USDA Economic Research Service and BMI and morality data from the World Health Organization.

19 *The End of Overeating:* David Kessler, *The End of Overeating: Taking Control of the Insatiable American Appetite* (New York: Macmillan, 2009).

19–20 **most other studies also show:** C. J. Lewis, Y. K. Park, P. B. Dexter, and E. A. Yetley, "Nutrient Intakes and Body Weights of Persons Consuming High and Moderate Levels of Added Sugars," *Journal of the American Dietetic Association* 92 (1992): 708–13. J. I. Macdiarmid, A. Vail, J. E. Cade, and J. E. Blundell, "The Sugar-Fat Relationship Revisited: Differences in Consumption between Men and Women of Varying BMI," *International Journal of Obesity* 22 (1998): 1053–61. C. Bolton-Smith, "Intake of Sugars in Relation to Fatness and Micronutrient Adequacy," *International Journal of Obesity* 20, suppl. 2 (1996): S31–33. J. O. Hill and A. M. Prentice, "Sugar and Body Weight Regulation," *American Journal of Clinical Nutrition* 62 (1995): 264S–74S. Wim H. M. Saris, "Sugars, Energy Metabolism, and Body Weight Control," *American Journal of Clinical Nutrition* 78 (2003): 850S–57S. S. H. Vermunt, W. J. Pasman, G. Schaafsma, and A. F. Kardinaal, "Effects of Sugar Intake on Body Weight: A Review," *Obesity Reviews* 4 (2003): 91–99. David Benton, "The Plausibility of Sugar Addiction and Its Role in Obesity and Eating Disorders," *Clinical Nutrition* 29 (2010): 288–303. M. A. van Baak and A. Astrup, "Consumption of Sugars and Body Weight," *Obesity Reviews* 10, suppl. 1 (2009): 9–23.

20 **studies have not found that it does:** K. J. Melanson, L. Zukley, J. Lowndes, V. Nguyen, T. J. Angelopoulos, J. M. Rippe, et al., "Effects of High-Fructose Corn Syrup and Sucrose Consumption on Circulating Glucose, Insulin, Leptin, and Ghrelin and on Appetite in Normal-Weight Women," *Nutrition* 23 (2007): 103–12. John S. White, "Straight Talk about High-Fructose Corn Syrup: What It Is and What It Ain't," *American Journal of Clinical Nutrition* 88 (2008): 1716S–21S.

20 **Gary Taubes:** See *Good Calories, Bad Calories* (New York: Alfred A. Knopf, 2007). Also: *Why We Get Fat and What to Do About It* (New York: Alfred A. Knopf, 2011).

22 **Stone Age ancestors had a diet with plenty of meat:** L. Cordain, S. B. Eaton, J. B. Miller, N. Mann, and K. Hill, "The Paradoxical Nature of Hunter-Gatherer Diets: Meat-Based, yet Non-Atherogenic," *European Journal of Clinical Nutrition* 56, suppl. 1 (2002): S42–52.

23 **more dairy food is linked to lower weights:** See Jasminka Z. Ilich, "A Lighter Side of Calcium: Role of Calcium and Dairy Foods in Body Weight," *Arhiv Za Higijenu Rada i Toksikologiju* 56 (2005): 33–38; G. C. Major, J. P. Chaput, M. Ledoux, S. St.-Pierre, G. H. Anderson, M. B. Zemel, and A. Tremblay, "Recent Developments in Calcium-Related Obesity Research," *Obesity Reviews* 9 (2008): 428–45; Marta Van Loan, "The Role of Dairy Foods and Dietary Calcium in Weight Management," *Journal of the American College of Nutrition* 28, suppl. 1 (2009): 120S–29S; Michael B. Zemel, "The Role of Dairy Foods in Weight Management," *Journal of the American College of Nutrition* 24 (2005): 537S–46S; Gianvincenzo Barba and Paola Russo, "Dairy Foods, Dietary Calcium and Obesity: A Short Review of the Evidence," *Nutrition Metabolism & Cardiovascular Diseases* 16 (2006): 445–51.

23 **vitamin D, which is also linked to lower weights:** See Elena Rodriguez-Rodriguez, Beatriz Navia, Ana M. Lopez-Sobaler, and Rosa M. Ortega, "Vitamin D in Overweight/Obese Women and Its Relationship with Dietetic and Anthropometric Variables," *Obesity* 17 (2009): 778–82; Y. J. Foss, "Vitamin D Deficiency Is the Cause of Common Obesity," *Medical Hypotheses* 72 (2009): 314–21.

23 **vitamin D levels have been falling:** Anne C. Looker, Christine M. Pfeiffer, David A. Lacher, Rosemary L. Schleicher, Mary Frances Picciano, and Elizabeth A. Yetley, "Serum 25-Hydroxyvitamin D Status of the US Population: 1988–1994 Compared with 2000–2004," *American Journal of Clinical Nutrition* 88 (2008): 1519–27.

25 **lower our *good* cholesterol:** T. W. de Bruin, C. B. Brouwer, M. van Linde-Sibenius Trip, H. Jansen, and D. W. Erkelens, "Different Postprandial Metabolism of Olive Oil and Soybean Oil: A Possible Mechanism of the High-Density Lipoprotein Conserving Effect of Olive Oil," *American Journal of Clinical Nutrition* 58 (1993): 477–83.

27 **trans fats have a measureable harmful effect:** Alberto Ascherio, "Trans Fatty Acids and Blood Lipids," *Atherosclerosis Supplements* 7 (2006): 25–27. Valentina Remig, Barry Franklin, Simeon Margolis, Georgia Kostas, Theresa Nece, and James C. Street, "Trans Fats in America: A Review of Their Use, Consumption, Health Implications, and Regulation," *Journal of the American Dietetic Association* 110 (2010): 585–92. Fred A. Kummerow, "The Negative Effects of Hydrogenated Trans Fats and What to Do About Them," *Atherosclerosis* 205 (2009): 458–65. Dariush Mozaffarian, Martijn B. Katan, Alberto Ascherio, Meir J. Stampfer, and Walter C. Willett, "Trans Fatty

Acids and Cardiovascular Disease," *New England Journal of Medicine* 354 (2006): 1601–13. D. Mozaffarian and R. Clarke, "Quantitative Effects on Cardiovascular Risk Factors and Coronary Heart Disease Risk of Replacing Partially Hydrogenated Vegetable Oils with Other Fats and Oils," *European Journal of Clinical Nutrition* 63, suppl. 2 (2009): S22–33.

27 **intentionally suppressed:** Mary Enig and Sally Fallon, "Oiling of America," *Nexus* 6/1–2 (1998–99). Available at www.drcranton.com /nutrition/oiling.htm.

27 **soybeans with very low levels of omega-3:** Kayla Hendrick, " 'Low-Lin' Oil Helps Keep Us Healthier and Profitable: New Enhanced-Trait Varieties to Help Soybean Oil Win Back Significant Share of the Market for Edible Oils," *Beyond the Bean* (2011). Monica Whent, Junjie Hao, Margaret Slavin, Martin Zhou, Jiuzhou Song, William Kenworthy, and Liangli Lucy Yu, "Effect of Genotype, Environment, and Their Interaction on Chemical Composition and Antioxidant Properties of Low-Linolenic Soybeans Grown in Maryland," *Journal of Agricultural & Food Chemistry* 57 (2009): 10163–74.

28 **thirty-two pounds of cooking oil:** H. Hiza, L. Bente, and T. Fungwe, "Nutrient Content of the U.S. Food Supply, 2005." *Home Economics Research Report* No. 28: Center for Nutrition Policy and Promotion, U.S. Department of Agriculture, 2008.

29 **researchers in Heidelberg:** Katharina Nimptsch, Gabriele Berg-Beckhoff, and Jakob Linseisen, "Effect of Dietary Fatty Acid Intake on Prospective Weight Change in the Heidelberg Cohort of the European Prospective Investigation into Cancer and Nutrition," *Public Health Nutrition* 13 (2010): 1636–46.

30 **obese adults and children have higher levels of linoleic:** See, for example, Martin Karlsson, S. Marild, J. Brandberg, L. Lonn, P. Friberg, and B. Strandik, "Serum Phospholipid Fatty Acids, Adipose Tissue and Metabolic Markers in Obese Adolescents," *Obesity* 14 (2006): 1931–39; Tamas Decsi, D. Molnar, and B. Koletzko, "Long-Chain Polyunsaturated Fatty Acids in Plasma Lipids of Obese Children," *Lipids* 31 (1996): 305–11; George V. Dedoussis, Alexandra Kapiri, Nick Kalogeropoulos, Anastasia Samara, Dimitris Dimitriadis, Daniel Lambert, et al., "Adipokine Expression in Adipose Tissue and in Peripheral Blood Mononuclear Cells in Children Correlation with BMI and Fatty Acid Content," *Clinica Chimica Acta* 410 (2009): 85–89; F. Massiera, P. Saint-Marc, J. Seydoux, T. Murata, T. Kobayashi, S. Narumiya, P. Guesnet, E. Z. Amri, R. Negrel, and G. Ailhaud, "Arachidonic Acid and Prostacyclin Signaling Promote Adipose Tissue Development: A Human Health Concern?" *Journal of Lipid Research* 44 (2003): 271–79; G. Fontani, F. Corradeschi, A. Felici, F. Alfatti, R. Bugarini, A. I. Fiaschi, et al., "Blood Profiles, Body Fat and Mood State in Healthy Subjects on Different Diets Supplemented with Omega-3 Polyunsaturated Fatty Acids," *European Journal of Clinical Investigation* 35 (2005): 499–507. See also p. 216.

30 **soybean oil also makes them gain weight:** See Gerard Ailhaud, F. Massiera, P. Weill, P. Legrand, J. M. Alessandri, and P. Guesnet, "Temporal Changes in Dietary Fats: Role of N-6 Polyunsaturated Fatty Acids in Excessive Adipose Tissue Development and Relationship to Obesity," *Progress in Lipid Research* 45 (2006): 203–36; D. A. Pan and L. H. Storlien, "Dietary Lipid Profile Is a Determinant of Tissue Phospholipid Fatty Acid Composition and Rate of Weight Gain in Rats," *Journal of Nutrition* 123 (1993): 512–19; Michael Pellizzon, A. Buison, F. Ordiz, Jr., L. S. Ana, and K. L. C. Jen, "Effects of Dietary Fatty Acids and Exercise on Body-Weight Regulation and Metabolism in Rats," *Obesity Research* 10 (2002): 947–55.

30 *gamma-tocopherol:* See M. Meydani, J. S. Cohn, J. B. Macauley, J. R. McNamara, J. B. Blumberg, and E. J. Schaefer, "Postprandial Changes in the Plasma Concentration of Alpha- and Gamma-Tocopherol in Human Subjects Fed a Fat-Rich Meal Supplemented with Fat-Soluble Vitamins," *Journal of Nutrition* 119 (1989): 1252–58. Also J. Lehmann, H. L. Martin, E. L. Lashley, M. W. Marshall, and J. T. Judd, "Vitamin E in Foods from High and Low Linoleic Acid Diets," *Journal of the American Dietetic Association* 86 (1986): 1208–16; L. Beth Dixon, Amy F. Subar, Louise Wideroff, Frances E. Thompson, Lisa L. Kahle, and Nancy Potischman, "Carotenoid and Tocopherol Estimates from the NCI Diet History Questionnaire Are Valid Compared with Multiple Recalls and Serum Biomarkers," *Journal of Nutrition* 136 (2006): 3054–61; L. M. Iakushuina, N. M. Lykova, and I. A. Ryndakova, "Direct Determination of Tocopherols in Plant Oils by High-Performance Liquid Chromatography," *Voprosy Pitaniia* (1987): 59–61; Sameera A. Talegawkar, Elizabeth J. Johnson, Teresa Carithers, Herman A. Taylor, Jr., Margaret L. Bogle, and Katherine L. Tucker, "Total Alpha-Tocopherol Intakes Are Associated with Serum Alpha-Tocopherol Concentrations in African American Adults," *Journal of Nutrition* 137 (2007): 2297–2303.

30 **soybean oil lowers HDL:** Z. Lu, S. Hendrich, N. Shen, P. J. White, and L. R. Cook, "Low Linolenate and Commercial Soybean Oils Diminish Serum HDL Cholesterol in Young Free-Living Adult Females," *Journal of the American College of Nutrition* 16 (1997): 562–69.

31 **trans fats and high omega-6 levels with larger waist:** Merethe H. Rokling-Andersen, Arild C. Rustan, Andreas J. Wensaas, Olav Kaalhus, Hege Wergedahl, Therese H. Ost, et al., "Marine N-3 Fatty Acids Promote Size Reduction of Visceral Adipose Depots, Without Altering Body Weight and Composition, in Male Wistar Rats Fed a High-Fat Diet," *British Journal of Nutrition* 102 (2009): 995–1006. J. O. Hill, J. C. Peters, D. Lin, F. Yakubu, H. Greene, and L. Swift, "Lipid Accumulation and Body Fat Distribution Is Influenced by Type of Dietary Fat Fed to Rats," *International Journal of Obesity* 17 (1993): 223–36. Mark Borkman, L. H. Storlien, D. A. Pan, A. B. Jenkins, D. J. Chisholm, and L. V. Campbell,

"The Relation Between Insulin Sensitivity and the Fatty-Acid Composition of Skeletal-Muscle Phospholipids," *New England Journal of Medicine* 328 (1993): 238–44. J. M. Fernandez-Real and W. Ricart, "Insulin Resistance and Inflammation in an Evolutionary Perspective: The Contribution of Cytokine Genotype/Phenotype to Thriftiness," *Diabetologia* 42 (1999): 1367–74. Shun Wang, Aiqun Ma, Shaowu Song, Qinghai Quan, Xinfeng Zhao, and Xiaohui Zheng, "Fasting Serum Free Fatty Acid Composition, Waist/Hip Ratio and Insulin Activity in Essential Hypertensive Patients," *Hypertension Research—Clinical & Experimental* 31 (2008): 623–32. S. B. Haugaard, A. Vaag, C. E. Hoy, and S. Madsbad, "Sex and Muscle Structural Lipids in Obese Subjects—an Impact on Insulin Action?" *European Journal of Clinical Investigation* 38 (2008): 494–501. E. Lee, S. Lee, and Y. Park, "N-3 Polyunsaturated Fatty Acids and Trans Fatty Acids in Patients with the Metabolic Syndrome: A Case-Control Study in Korea," *British Journal of Nutrition* 100 (2008): 609–14.

31 **Eicosanoids made from arachidonic:** Y. Fujitani, K. Aritake, Y. Kanaoka, T. Goto, N. Takahashi, K. Fujimori, and T. Kawada, "Pronounced Adipogenesis and Increased Insulin Sensitivity Caused by Overproduction of Prostaglandin D2 in Vivo," *FEBS Journal* 277 (2010): 1410–19.

32 **endocannabinoids also stimulate our appetites:** Vincenzo Di Marzo and Isabel Matias, "Endocannabinoid Control of Food Intake and Energy Balance," *Nature Neuroscience* 8 (2005): 585–89. H. S. Hansen and A. Artmann, "Endocannabinoids and Nutrition," *Journal of Neuroendocrinology* 20, suppl. 1 (2008): 94–99. Kathy Keenan Isoldi and Louis J. Aronne, "The Challenge of Treating Obesity: The Endocannabinoid System as a Potential Target," *Journal of the American Dietetic Association* 108 (2008): 823–31.

32 **Higher levels of endocannabinoids are found in obese:** M. Bluher, S. Engeli, N. Kloting, J. Berndt, M. Fasshauer, S. Batkai, P. Pacher, M. R. Schon, J. Jordan, and M. Stumvoll, "Dysregulation of the Peripheral and Adipose Tissue Endocannabinoid System in Human Abdominal Obesity," *Diabetes* 55 (2006): 3053–60. M. Cote, I. Matias, I. Lemieux, S. Petrosino, N. Almeras, J. P. Despres, and Marzo V. Di, "Circulating Endocannabinoid Levels, Abdominal Adiposity and Related Cardiometabolic Risk Factors in Obese Men," *International Journal of Obesity* 31 (2007): 692–99.

32 **make much more appetite-stimulating endocannabinoid:** Isabel Matias, Gianfranca Carta, Elisabetta Murru, Stefania Petrosino, Sebastiano Banni, and Vincenzo Di Marzo, "Effect of Polyunsaturated Fatty Acids on Endocannabinoid and N-Acyl-Ethanolamine Levels in Mouse Adipocytes," *Biochimica et Biophysica Acta* 1781 (2008): 52–60. Andreas Artmann, Gitte Petersen, Lars I. Hellgren, Julie Boberg, Christian Skonberg, Christine Nellemann, Steen Honore Hansen, and Harald S. Hansen, "Influence of Dietary Fatty Acids on Endocannabinoid and N-Acylethanolamine Levels in Rat Brain, Liver and Small Intestine," *Biochimica et Biophysica Acta* 1781 (2008): 200–212.

33 **more omega-3 and less omega-6 in their blood and diet weigh**
    less: Michelle Micallef, Irene Munro, Melinda Phang, and Manohar
    Garg, "Plasma N-3 Polyunsaturated Fatty Acids Are Negatively Associ-
    ated with Obesity," *British Journal of Nutrition* 102 (2009): 1370–74. Yukio
    Yamori, "Worldwide Epidemic of Obesity: Hope for Japanese Diets,"
    Clinical & Experimental Pharmacology & Physiology 31, suppl. 2 (2004): S2–4.
    A. Elizondo, J. Araya, R. Rodrigo, J. Poniachik, A. Csendes, F. Malu-
    enda, J. C. Diaz, C. Signorini, C. Sgherri, M. Comporti, and L. A.
    Videla, "Polyunsaturated Fatty Acid Pattern in Liver and Erythrocyte
    Phospholipids from Obese Patients," *Obesity* 15 (2007): 24–31. Martin
    Karlsson, S. Marild, J. Brandberg, L. Lonn, P. Friberg, and B. Strandik,
    "Serum Phospholipid Fatty Acids, Adipose Tissue and Metabolic Markers
    in Obese Adolescents," *Obesity* 14 (2006): 1931–39. Carine Klein-Platat, J.
    Davis, M. Oujaa, J. L. Schleinger, and C. Simon, "Plasma Fatty Acid
    Composition Is Associated with the Metabolic Syndrome and Low-Grade
    Inflammation in Overweight Adolescents," *American Journal of Clinical
    Nutrition* 82 (2005): 1178–84. Tamas Decsi, D. Molnar, and B. Koletzko,
    "Long-Chain Polyunsaturated Fatty Acids in Plasma Lipids of Obese
    Children," *Lipids* 31 (1996): 305–11. E. H. Moriguchi, Y. Moriguchi, and
    Y. Yamori, "Impact of Diet on the Cardiovascular Risk Profile of Japanese
    Immigrants Living in Brazil: Contributions of World Health Organiza-
    tion Cardiac and Monalisa Studies," *Clinical & Experimental Pharmacology &
    Physiology* 31, suppl. 2 (2004): S5–7. S. Scaglioni, E. Verduci, M. Salvioni,
    M. G. Bruzzese, G. Radaelli, R. Zetterstrom, E. Riva, and C. Agostoni,
    "Plasma Long-Chain Fatty Acids and the Degree of Obesity in Italian
    Children," *Acta Paediatrica Scandinavica* 95 (2006): 964–69. Scott A. Sands,
    Kimberly J. Reid, Sheryl L. Windsor, and William S. Harris, "The
    Impact of Age, Body Mass Index, and Fish Intake on the EPA and DHA
    Content of Human Erythrocytes," *Lipids* 40 (2005): 343–47. S. B.
    Haugaard, A. Vaag, C. E. Hoy, and S. Madsbad, "Sex and Muscle Struc-
    tural Lipids in Obese Subjects—an Impact on Insulin Action?" *European
    Journal of Clinical Investigation* 38 (2008): 494–501. See p. 216.
33 **omega-3 in the diet helps women to lose weight:** Alison M. Hill,
    J. D. Buckley, K. J. Murphy, and P. R. C. Howe, "Combining Fish-Oil
    Supplements with Regular Aerobic Exercise Improves Body Composition
    and Cardiovascular Disease Risk Factors," *American Journal of Clinical
    Nutrition* 85 (2007): 1267–74. M. Kunesova, R. Braunerova, P. Hlavaty,
    E. Tvrzicka, B. Stankova, J. Skrha, et al., "The Influence of N-3 Polyunsat-
    urated Fatty Acids and Very Low Calorie Diet During a Short-Term
    Weight Reducing Regimen on Weight Loss and Serum Fatty Acid Com-
    position in Severely Obese Women," *Physiological Research* 55 (2006): 63–72.
    Morvarid Kabir, Geraldine Skurnik, Nadia Naour, Valeria Pechtner,
    Emmanuelle Meugnier, Sophie Rome, et al., "Treatment for 2 Months
    with N-3 Polyunsaturated Fatty Acids Reduces Adiposity," *American Journal*

of Clinical Nutrition 86 (2007): 1670–79. Kentaro Matsumura, "Effects of Eicosapentaenoic Acid on Visceral Fat and Heart Rate Variability: Assessment by Power Spectral Analysis," *Journal of Cardiology* 50 (2007): 243–51.

33 **Animals fed more omega-3 and less omega-6:** J. J. D. Buckley and P. R. C. Howe, "Anti-Obesity Effects of Long-Chain Omega-3 Polyunsaturated Fatty Acids," *Obesity Reviews* 10 (2009): 648–59. Ruzickova, M. Rossmeisl, T. Prazak, P. Flachs, J. Sponarova, M. Veck, E. Tvrzicka, M. Bryhn, and J. Kopecky, "Omega-3 PUFA of Marine Origin Limit Diet-Induced Obesity in Mice by Reducing Cellularity of Adipose Tissue," *Lipids* 39 (2004): 1177–85. H. Wang, L. H. Storlien, and X. F. Huang, "Effects of Dietary Fat Types on Body Fatness, Leptin, and ARC Leptin Receptor, NPY, and AGRP MRNA Expression," *American Journal of Physiology* 282 (2002): E1352–59. Bungo Shirouchi, Koji Nagao, Nao Inoue, Takeshi Ohkubo, Hidehiko Hibino, and Teruyoshi Yanagita, "Effect of Dietary Omega 3 Phosphatidylcholine on Obesity-Related Disorders in Obese Otsuka Long-Evans Tokushima Fatty Rats," *Journal of Agricultural & Food Chemistry* 55 (2007): 7170–76. Takuya Mori, Hidehiko Kondo, Tadashi Hase, Ichiro Tokimitsu, and Takatoshi Murase, "Dietary Fish Oil Upregulates Intestinal Lipid Metabolism and Reduces Body Weight Gain in C57bl/6j Mice," *Journal of Nutrition* 137 (2007): 2629–34.

33 **omega-3 fat also has the opposite effect on the waist:** Francoise Belzung, T. Raclot, and R. Groscolas, "Fish Oil N-3 Fatty Acids Selectively Limit the Hypertrophy of Abdominal Fat Depots in Growing Rats Fed High-Fat Diets," *American Journal of Physiology* 264 (1993): R1111–18. H. Moriya, M. Hosokawa, and K. Miyashita, "Combination Effect of Herring Roe Lipids and Proteins on Plasma Lipids and Abdominal Fat Weight of Mouse," *Journal of Food Science* 72 (2007): C231–34. A. Ghosh, "Comparison of Anthropometric, Metabolic and Dietary Fatty Acids Profiles in Lean and Obese Dyslipidaemic Asian Indian Male Subjects," *European Journal of Clinical Nutrition* 61 (2007): 412–19. Shun Wang, Aiqun Ma, Shaowu Song, Qinghai Quan, Xinfeng Zhao, and Xiaohui Zheng, "Fasting Serum Free Fatty Acid Composition, Waist/Hip Ratio and Insulin Activity in Essential Hypertensive Patients," Hypertension Research— Clinical & Experimental 31 (2008): 623–32.

33 **Omega-3 helps to reduce weight:** B. Dziedzic, J. Szemraj, J. Bartkowiak, and A. Walczewska, "Various Dietary Fats Differentially Change the Gene Expression of Neuropeptides Involved in Body Weight Regulation in Rats," Journal of Neuroendocrinology 19 (2007): 364–73. P. Flachs, V. Mohamed-Ali, O. Horakova, M. Rossmeisl, M. J. Hosseinzadeh-Attar, M. Hensler, J. Ruzickova, and J. Kopecky, "Polyunsaturated Fatty Acids of Marine Origin Upregulate Mitochondrial Biogenesis and Induce Beta-Oxidation in White Fat," Diabetologia 48 (2005): 2365–75. R. A. Baillie, R. Takada, M. Nakamura, and S. D. Clarke, "Coordinate Induction of Peroxisomal Acyl-CoA Oxidase and UCP-3 by Dietary Fish Oil: A

Mechanism for Decreased Body Fat Deposition," *Prostaglandins Leukotrienes & Essential Fatty Acids* 60 (1999): 351–56.

33 **appetite, omega-3 reduces it:** Dolores Parra, Alfons Ramel, Narcisa Bandarra, Mairead Kiely, J. Alfredo Martinez, and Inga Thorsdottir, "A Diet Rich in Long Chain Omega-3 Fatty Acids Modulates Satiety in Overweight and Obese Volunteers during Weight Loss," *Appetite* 51 (2008): 676–80.

33 **least hungry after meals high in omega-3:** J. C. Lovejoy, M. M. Most, C. M. Champagne, L. de Jonge, G. A. Bray, S. R. Smith, et al., "Different Fatty Acids Differentially Affect Hunger Ratings in Obese Adults," *Obesity Research* 9, suppl. 3 (2001): 122S.

33 **Omega-3 fats also reduce the amount of insulin:** S. O. Ebbesson, P. M. Risica, L. O. Ebbesson, J. M. Kennish, and M. E. Tejero, "Omega-3 Fatty Acids Improve Glucose Tolerance and Components of the Metabolic Syndrome in Alaskan Eskimos: The Alaska Siberia Project," *International Journal of Circumpolar Health* 64 (2005): 396–408.

33 **less omega-3 in the blood:** See Margit Kornsteiner, Ingrid Singer, and Ibrahim Elmadfa, "Very Low N-3 Long-Chain Polyunsaturated Fatty Acid Status in Austrian Vegetarians and Vegans," *Annals of Nutrition & Metabolism* 52 (2008): 37–47; Patrick Rump and G. Hornstra, "The N-3 and N-6 Polyunsaturated Fatty Acid Composition of Plasma Phospholipids in Pregnant Women and Their Infants: Relation with Maternal Linoleic Acid Intake," *Clinical Chemistry and Laboratory Medicine* 40 (2002): 32–39.

34 **Our Stone Age ancestors:** Remko S. Kuipers, Martine F. Luxwold, D. A. Janneke Dijck-Brouwer, S. Boyd Eaton, Michael A. Crawford, Loren Cordain, and Frits A. J. Muskiet, "Estimated Macronutrient and Fatty Acid Intakes from an East African Paleolithic Diet," *British Journal of Nutrition* 104 (2010): 1666–87.

34 **Michael Pollan:** *The Omnivore's Dilemma: A Natural History of Four Meals* (New York: Penguin Press, 2006).

34 **Naturally grass-fed animals:** Cynthia A. Daley, Amber Abbott, Patrick S. Doyle, Glenn A. Nader, and Stephanie Larson, "A Review of Fatty Acid Profiles and Antioxidant Content in Grass-Fed and Grain-Fed Beef," *Nutrition Journal* 9 (2010): 10. P. Legrand, B. Schmitt, J. Mourot, D. Catheline, G. Chesneau, M. Mireaux, N. Kerhoas, and P. Weill, "The Consumption of Food Products from Linseed-Fed Animals Maintains Erythrocyte Omega-3 Fatty Acids in Obese Humans," *Lipids* 45 (2010): 11–19.

35 **chickens have also been switched over to corn-based feed:** Y. Wang, C. Lehane, K. Ghebremeskel, M. A. Crawford, Yiqun Wang, Catherine Lehane, et al., "Modern Organic and Broiler Chickens Sold for Human Consumption Provide More Energy from Fat than Protein," *Public Health Nutrition* 13 (2010): 400–408.

35 **most farmed fish have more omega-6:** Kelly L. Weaver, Priscilla Ivester, Joshua A. Chilton, Martha D. Wilson, Prativa Pandey, and Floyd H. Chilton, "The Content of Favorable and Unfavorable Polyunsaturated Fatty Acids Found in Commonly Eaten Fish," *Journal of the American Dietetic Association* 108 (2008): 1178–85.

35 **the omega-3 it contains is no longer available:** H. Chung, J. A. Nettleton, R. N. Lemaitre, R. G. Barr, M. Y. Tsai, R. P. Tracy, et al., "Frequency and Type of Seafood Consumed Influence Plasma (N-3) Fatty Acid Concentrations," *Journal of Nutrition* 138 (2008): 2422–27. M. I. Gladyshev, G. A. Gubanenko, N. N. Sushchik, S. M. Demirchieva, and G. S. Kalacheva, "Influence of Different Methods of Cooking of Hunchback Salmon on Contents of Polyunsaturated Fatty Acids," *Voprosy Pitaniia* 75 (2006): 47–50.

36 **our consumption of the health-promoting monounsaturated fats:** A. Keys, A. Menotti, M. J. Karvonen, C. Aravanis, H. Blackburn, R. Buzina, B. S. Djordjevic, A. S. Dontas, F. Fidanza, M. H. Keys, et al., "The Diet and 15-Year Death Rate in the Seven Countries Study," *American Journal of Epidemiology* 124 (1986): 903–15. Vincenzo Solfrizzi, Alessia D'Introno, Anna M. Colacicco, Cristiano Capurso, et al., "Unsaturated Fatty Acids Intake and All-Causes Mortality: A 8.5-Year Follow-Up of the Italian Longitudinal Study on Aging," *Experimental Gerontology* 40 (2005): 335–43.

37 **smoking accounting for more than *90 percent* of the changes:** Cigarettes per capita explain 91 percent of the *increase* in age-adjusted heart disease death rates in American men from 1900 to 1963 and 94 percent of the *decrease* from 1964 to 2006.

37 **what we would expect if smoking were the cause:** See the differences between smokers and nonsmokers in J. Stamler, D. Wentworth, and J. D. Neaton, "Is Relationship Between Serum Cholesterol and Risk of Premature Death from Coronary Heart Disease Continuous and Graded?" *Journal of the American Medical Association* 256 (1986): 2823–28. Ancel Keys, *Seven Countries* (Cambridge, Mass: Harvard University Press, 1980).

37 **women's smoking rates:** American Lung Association, "Trends in Tobacco Use," February 2010, www.lungusa.org/finding-cures/our-research/trend-reports/Tobacco-Trend-Report.pdf.

42 **mental furniture comes from our culture:** See Steven Pinker, *The Blank Slate: The Modern Denial of Human Nature* (New York: Viking, 2002).

42 **David Buss:** David M. Buss, "Sex Differences in Human Mate Preferences: Evolutionary Hypothesis Tested in 37 Cultures," *Behavioral and Brain Sciences* 12 (1989): 1–49.

46 *no difference* **in the waist-hip ratios:** M. H. A. van Hooff, E. J. Voorhorst, M. B. H. Kaptein, and R. A. Hirasing, "Endocrine Features of

Polycystic Ovary Syndrome in a Random Population Sample of 14–16 Year Old Adolescents," *Human Reproduction* 14 (1999): 2223–29. Marcel H. A. Van Hooff, Feja J. Voorhorst, Margriet B. H. Kaptein, Remy A. Hirasing, Corrie Koppenaal, and Joop Schoemaker, "Polycystic Ovaries in Adolescents and the Relationship with Menstrual Cycle Patterns, Luteinizing Hormone, Androgens, and Insulin," *Fertility & Sterility* 74 (2000): 49–58.

47 **5 percent of their body weight:** Caroline M. Pond and Christine A. Mattacks, "The Anatomy of Adipose Tissue in Captive Macaca Monkeys and Its Implications for Human Biology," *Folia Primatol* 48 (1987): 164–85.

47 **preferred women with large or fat legs:** Peter J. Brown and Melvin Konner, "An Anthropological Perspective on Obesity," *Annals of the New York Academy of Science* 499 (1987): 29–46.

47 **fed extra food:** See, for example, Rebecca Popenoe, *Feeding Desire: Fatness, Beauty, and Sexuality Among a Saharan People* (New York: Routledge, 2004).

47 **R. Matthew Montoya:** "Gender Similarities and Differences in Preferences for Specific Body Parts," *Current Research in Social Psychology* 13 (2007): 133–44. See also Robert W. Wildman, A. Brown, and C. Trice, "Note on Males' and Females' Preferences for Opposite Sex Body Parts, Bust Sizes, and Bust-Revealing Clothes," *Psychological Reports* 38 (1976): 485–86.

48 **costs about sixty thousand extra calories to have a baby:** This does not include the calories used to store more fat. See Nancy F. Butte and J. C. King, "Energy Requirements During Pregnancy and Lactation," *Public Health Nutrition* 8 (2005): 1010–27.

49 **a mother's lower-body fat will go down:** See our paper "Changes in Body Fat Distribution in Relation to Parity in American Women: A Covert Form of Maternal Depletion," *American Journal of Physical Anthropology* 131 (2006): 295–302.

50 **nerve cells to grow:** See Sheila M. Innis, "Dietary Omega 3 Fatty Acids and the Developing Brain," *Brain Research* 1237 (2008): 35–43; Frances Calderon and Hee-Yong Kim, "Docosahexaenoic Acid Promotes Neurite Growth in Hippocampal Neurons," *Journal of Neurochemistry* 90 (2004): 979–88; P. Green, S. Glozman, B. Kamensky, and B. Yavin, "Developmental Changes in Rat Membrane Lipids and Fatty Acids: The Preferential Prenatal Accumulation of Docosahexaenoic Acid," *Journal of Lipid Research* 40 (1999): 960–66; N. Auestad and S. M. Innis, "Dietary N-3 Fatty Acid Restriction During Gestation in Rats: Neuronal Cell Body and Growth-Cone Fatty Acids," *American Journal of Clinical Nutrition* 71 (2000): 312S–14S; Klara Kitajka, L. G. Puskas, A. Zvara, L. Hackler, Jr., G. Barcelo-Coblijn, Y. K. Yoo, and T. Farkas, "The Role of N-3 Polyunsaturated Fatty Acids in Brain: Modulation of Rat Brain Gene Expression

by Dietary N-3 Fatty Acids," *Proceedings of the National Academy of Sciences* 99 (2002): 2619–24.

50 **send messages:** Nigel Turner, P. L. Else, and A. J. Hulbert, "Docosahexaenoic Acid (DHA) Content of Membranes Determines Molecular Activity of the Sodium Pump: Implications for Disease States and Metabolism," *Naturwissenshaften* 90 (2003): 521–23. Also: J. M. Bourre, M. Francois, A. Youyou, O. Dumont, M. Piciotti, G. Pascal, and G. Durand, "The Effects of Dietary Alpha-Linolenic Acid on the Composition of Nerve Membranes, Enzymatic Activity, Amplitude of Electrophysiological Parameters, Resistance to Poisons and Performance of Learning Tasks in Rats," *Journal of Nutrition* 119 (1989): 1880–92; S. Yoshida, A. Yasuda, H. Kawazato, K. Sakai, T. Shimada, M. Takeshita, S. Yuasa, T. Kobayashi, S. Watanabe, and H. Okuyama, "Synaptic Vesicle Ultrastructural Changes in the Rat Hippocampus Induced by a Combination of Alpha-Linolenate Deficiency and a Learning Task," *Journal of Neurochemistry* 68 (1997): 1261–68. And: Fernando Gomez-Pinilla, "Brain Foods: The Effects of Nutrients on Brain Function," *Nature Reviews Neurosciences* 9 (2008): 568–78. For DHA's effect on the production of neurotransmitters, see H. Li, D. Liu, and E. Zhang, "Effect of Fish Oil Supplementation on Fatty Acid Composition and Neurotransmitters of Growing Rats," *Journal of Hygiene Research* 29 (2000): 47–49; S. de la Presa Owens and S. M. Innis, "Docosahexaenoic and Arachidonic Acid Prevent a Decrease in Dopaminergic and Serotoninergic Neurotransmitters in Frontal Cortex Caused by a Linoleic and Alpha-Linolenic Acid Deficient Diet in Formula-Fed Piglets," *Journal of Nutrition* 129 (1999): 2088–93.

50 **thousands of connections:** R. J. Wurtman, M. Cansev, and I. H. Ulus, "Synapse Formation Is Enhanced by Oral Administration of Uridine and DHA, the Circulating Precursors of Brain Phosphatides," *Journal of Nutrition, Health & Aging* 13 (2009): 189–97. M. Cansev and R. J. Wurtman, "Chronic Administration of Docosahexaenoic Acid or Eicosapentaenoic Acid, but Not Arachidonic Acid, Alone or in Combination with Uridine, Increases Brain Phosphatide and Synaptic Protein Levels in Gerbils," *Neuroscience* 148 (2007): 421–31. Lesley G. Robson, Simon Dyall, David Sidloff, and Adina T. Michael-Titus, "Omega-3 Polyunsaturated Fatty Acids Increase the Neurite Outgrowth of Rat Sensory Neurones Throughout Development and in Aged Animals," *Neurobiology of Aging* 31 (2010): 678–87. DHA also turns on genes in the brain: Klara Kitajka, L. G. Puskas, A. Zvara, L. Hackler, Jr., G. Barcelo-Coblijn, Y. K. Yoo, and T. Farkas, "The Role of N-3 Polyunsaturated Fatty Acids in Brain: Modulation of Rat Brain Gene Expression by Dietary N-3 Fatty Acids," *Proceedings of the National Academy of Sciences* 99 (2002): 2619–24.

50 **five football or soccer fields:** The membrane surface area of a typical neuron is 250,000 square micrometers: M. F. Bear, B. W. Connors, and

M. A. Paradiso, *Neuroscience: Exploring the Brain*, 2nd ed. (Baltimore: Lippincott Williams and Wilkins, 2001), 97. For 100 billion neurons this amounts to 25,000 square meters or 270,000 square feet.

50 **DHA is much harder to come by:** We may all be descended from humans who lived by the sea and ate shellfish rich in omega-3: see Curtis W. Marean, "When the Sea Saved Humanity," *Scientific American* 303 (2) (August 2010): 55–61.

50 **babies fed either breast milk or formula with added DHA do better:** See Joyce C. McCann and B. N. Ames, "Is Docosahexaenoic Acid, an N-3 Long-Chain Polyunsaturated Fatty Acid, Required for Development of Normal Brain Function? An Overview of Evidence from Cognitive and Behavioral Tests in Humans and Animals," *American Journal of Clinical Nutrition* 82 (2005): 281–95. Also Jean-Marc Alessandri, Philippe Guesnet, Sylvie Vancassel, Pierre Astorg, Isabelle Denis, Benedicte Langelier, Sabah Aid, et al., "Polyunsaturated Fatty Acids in the Central Nervous System: Evolution of Concepts and Nutritional Implications Throughout Life," *Reproduction, Nutrition, Development* 44 (2004): 509–38. Children that nurse longer also do better: Erik Lykke Mortensen, Kim Fleischer Michaelsen, Stephanie A. Sanders, and June Machover Reinisch, "The Association Between Duration of Breastfeeding and Adult Intelligence," *Journal of the American Medical Association* 287 (2002): 2365–71.

50 **children also do better on mental tests:** See Joshua T. Cohen, David C. Bellinger, William E. Connor, and Bennett A. Shaywitz, "A Quantitative Analysis of Prenatal Intake of N-3 Polyunsaturated Fatty Acids and Cognitive Development," *American Journal of Preventive Medicine* 29 (2005): 366–74.

50 **In our own research:** William D. Lassek and Steven J. C. Gaulin, "Sex Differences in the Influence of Dietary Fatty Acids on Cognition in Children." Presented at the *Human Behavior and Evolution Society* meeting in Kyoto, Japan, June 2007.

51 **ideally at least five drops (250 milligrams):** See Artemis P. Simopoulos, L. Leaf, and N. Salem, Jr., "Workshop on the Essentiality of and Recommended Dietary Intakes for Omega-6 and Omega-3 Fatty Acids," *Journal of the American College of Nutrition* 18 (1999): 487–89. The International Society for the Study of Fatty Acids and Lipids recommends at least 250 milligrams a day for adults: www.issfal.org/index.php?option=com _content&task=view&id=23&Itemid=8.

51 **DHA is quite scarce in our diet:** We can also make some DHA from the linolenic in our diet, but the process is very inefficient. See Melanie Plourde and Stephen C. Cunnane, "Extremely Limited Synthesis of Long Chain Polyunsaturates in Adults: Implications for Their Dietary Essentiality and Use as Supplements," *Applied Physiology, Nutrition, & Metabolism* 32 (2007): 619–34.

51 **just 70 milligrams of DHA in her daily diet:** Dietary DHA for the average American woman is 74 milligrams a day based on NHANES 2003–6. USDA estimates are 90 milligrams of DHA in the food supply: Shirley Gerrior, L. Bente and H. Hiza, *Nutrient Content of the U.S. Food Supply, 1909–2000*, Home Economics Research Report No. 56., U.S. Department of Agriculture, Center for Nutrition Policy and Promotion (2004).

51 **comes from her lower-body fat:** About 80 percent of the DHA and other essential fatty acids in a mother's milk comes from her fat: Thorsten U. Sauerwald, H. Demmelmair, N. Fidler, and B. Koletzko, "Polyunsaturated Fatty Acid Supply with Human Milk," *Advances in Experimental Medicine and Biology* 478 (2000): 261–70. The same is true in pregnancy: P. Haggarty, "Effect of Placental Function on Fatty Acid Requirements During Pregnancy," *European Journal of Clinical Nutrition* 58 (2004): 1559–70.

51 **fat that has much more DHA:** S. D. Phinney, J. S. Stern, K. E. Burke, A. B. Tang, G. Miller, and R. T. Holman, "Human Subcutaneous Adipose Tissue Shows Site-Specific Differences in Fatty Acid Composition," *American Journal of Clinical Nutrition* 60 (1994): 725–29. Maria Garaulet, F. Perez-Llamas, M. Perez-Ayala, P. Martinez, F. S. de Medina, F. J. Tebar, and S. Zamora, "Site-Specific Differences in the Fatty Acid Composition of Abdominal Adipose Tissue in an Obese Population from a Mediterranean Area," *American Journal of Clinical Nutrition* 74 (2001): 585–91. Shun Wang, Aiqun Ma, Shaowu Song, Qinghai Quan, Xinfeng Zhao, and Xiaohui Zheng, "Fasting Serum Free Fatty Acid Composition, Waist/Hip Ratio and Insulin Activity in Essential Hypertensive Patients," *Hypertension Research—Clinical & Experimental* 31 (2008): 623–32.

51 **begin dissolving some of her lower-body fat:** Marielle Rebuffe-Scrive, L. Enk, N. Crona, P. Lonnroth, L. Abrahamsson, U. Smith, and P. Bjorntorp, "Fat Cell Metabolism in Different Regions in Women: Effect of Menstrual Cycle, Pregnancy and Lactation," *Journal of Clinical Investigation* 75 (1985): 1973–76.

52 **special ability to transport DHA:** Fabienne L. Hanebutt, Hans Demmelmair, Barbara Schiessl, Elvira Larque, and Berthold Koletzko, "Long-Chain Polyunsaturated Fatty Acid (LC-PUFA) Transfer across the Placenta," *Clinical Nutrition* 27 (2008): 685–93.

52 **One pound of a mother's lower-body fat:** Fat from the buttocks has about 0.4 percent DHA: A. S. Biong, M. B. Veierod, D. S. Thelle, and J. I. Pedersen, "Intake of Milk Fat, Reflected in Adipose Tissue Fatty Acids and Risk of Myocardial Infarction: A Case-Control Study," *European Journal of Clinical Nutrition* 60 (2006): 236–44.

52 **typical nursing mother:** Nancy F. Butte, C. Garza, J. E. Stuff, E. O. Smith, and B. L. Nichols, "Effect of Maternal Diet and Body Composition on Lactational Performance," *American Journal of Clinical Nutrition* 39 (1984): 296–306.

52 **more fat than a newborn boy:** A. M. Guihard-Costa, E. Papiernik, G. Grange, and A. Richard, "Gender Differences in Neonatal Subcutaneous Fat Store in Late Gestation in Relation to Maternal Weight Gain," *Annals of Human Biology* 29 (2002): 26–36.

52 **girls (and women) also have a greater ability:** Erik J. Giltay, L. J. G. Gooren, A. W. F. T. Toorians, M. B. Katan, and P. L. Zock, "Docosa-hexaenoic Acid Concentrations Are Higher in Women Than in Men Because of Estrogenic Effects," *American Journal of Clinical Nutrition* 80 (2004): 1167–74.

52 **higher levels of DHA in their own brains:** Robert K. McNamara, Ronald Jandacek, Therese Rider, Patrick Tso, Yogesh Dwivedi, Rosa-linda C. Roberts, Robert R. Conley, and Ghanshyam N. Pandey, "Fatty Acid Composition of the Postmortem Prefrontal Cortex of Adolescent Male and Female Suicide Victims," *Prostaglandins Leukotrienes & Essential Fatty Acids* 80 (2009): 19–26.

53 **it is usually protected:** Marielle Rebuffe-Scrive, L. Enk, N. Crona, P. Lonnroth, L. Abrahamsson, U. Smith, and P. Bjorntorp, "Fat Cell Metabolism in Different Regions in Women: Effect of Menstrual Cycle, Pregnancy and Lactation," *Journal of Clinical Investigation* 75 (1985): 1973–76.

53 **Girls with more lower-body fat do mature earlier:** See our paper "Menarche Is Related to Fat Distribution," *American Journal of Physical Anthropology* 133 (2007):1147–51.

53 **scored better on the tests:** See our paper "Waist-Hip Ratio and Cogni-tive Ability: Is Gluteofemoral Fat a Privileged Store?" *Evolution and Human Behavior* 29 (2008): 26–34.

54 **more omega-3 fat in their blood:** See Shun Wang, Aiqun Ma, Shaowu Song, Qinghai Quan, Xinfeng Zhao, and Xiaohui Zheng, "Fast-ing Serum Free Fatty Acid Composition, Waist/Hip Ratio and Insulin Activity in Essential Hypertensive Patients," *Hypertension Research— Clinical & Experimental* 31 (2008): 623–32.

54 **DHA in her blood tends to decrease with each pregnancy:** M. D. M. Al, A. C. van Houwelingen, and G. Hornstra, "Long-Chain Polyun-saturated Fatty Acids, Pregnancy, and Pregnancy Outcome," *American Journal of Clinical Nutrition* 71, suppl. 1 (2000): S285–91.

54 **woman's brain can even shrink during her pregnancy:** Angela Oat-ridge, A. Holdcroft, N. Saeed, J. V. Hajnal, B. K. Puri, L. Fusi, and G. M. Bydder, "Change in Brain Size During and After Pregnancy: Study in Healthy Women and Women with Preeclampsia," *American Journal of Neu-roradiology* 23 (2002): 19–26.

59 **students actually have larger bust sizes:** Playmates' busts are larger than would be expected for women with BMIs and waist sizes as low as theirs.

60 **we measured the width of the waist and hip:** To see how the waist-hip ratio based on on the width of the waist and hip in an image or photograph

compares with the ratio based on waist and hip circumferences, we used the student sample and found that the waist–hip ratios calculated from their widths in a photograph are very similar to the ratios when the circumferences are measured.

60 **lights up the same pleasure centers:** Steven M. Platek and Devendra Singh, "Optimal Waist-to-Hip Ratios in Women Activate Neural Reward Centers in Men," *PLoS ONE* 5(2): E9042 (2010).

61 **eight thousand American women of all ages:** Women were asked for their low weight after eighteen in the NHANES I 1971–75 and also in the NHANES 1999–2000.

62 *less* **fertile, and** *less* **able to conceive children:** See, for example, G. W. Bates, S. R. Bates, and N. S. Whitworth, "Reproductive Failure in Women Who Practice Weight Control," *Fertility & Sterility* 37 (1982): 373–78. Francisco Bolumar, J. Olsen, M. Rebagliato, I. Saez-Lioret, and L. Bisanti, "Body Mass Index and Delayed Conception: A European Multicenter Study on Infertility and Subfecundity," *American Journal of Epidemiology* 151 (2000): 1072–79.

62 **Women athletes or ballet dancers:** Rose E. Frisch, "Body Fat, Puberty and Fertility," *Biological Reviews* 59 (1984): 161–88.

64 **Fatimata Ataher:** Fatimata's story is from Rachel Louise Snyder, "Shunned and Scarred for Life: Can the World's Most Helpless Female Outcasts Be Saved?" *Glamour*, February 2005.

64 **accounts for most of these deaths:** M. Nkata, "Maternal Mortality Due to Obstructed Labor," *International Journal of Gynaecology & Obstetrics* 57 (1997): 65–66. A. Rosenfield, "Maternal Mortality in Developing Countries: An Ongoing but Neglected 'Epidemic,'" *Journal of the American Medical Association* 262 (1989): 376–79. F. C. Vork, S. Kyanamina, and J. van Roosmalen, "Maternal Mortality in Rural Zambia," *Acta Obstetricia et Gynecologica Scandinavica* 76 (1997): 646–50. O. Frost, "Maternal and Perinatal Deaths in an Addis Ababa Hospital, 1980," *Ethiopian Medical Journal* 22 (1984): 143–46.

64 **few of their babies are born alive:** Bolajoko O. Olusanya and Olumuyiwa A. Solanke, "Predictors of Term Stillbirths in an Inner-City Maternity Hospital in Lagos, Nigeria," *Acta Obstetricia et Gynecologica Scandinavica* 88 (2009): 1243–51. Nazli Hossain, Nazeer Khan, and Nusrat H. Khan, "Obstetric Causes of Stillbirth at Low Socioeconomic Settings," *Journal of the Pakistan Medical Association* 59 (2009): 744–47.

64 **Many of the babies that are born alive:** J. van Roosmalen, "Birth Weights in Two Rural Hospitals in the United Republic of Tanzania," *Bulletin of the World Health Organization* 66 (1988): 653–58. T. Kandasamy, M. Merialdi, R. J. Guidotti, A. P. Betran, J. Harris-Requejo, F. Hakimi, P. F. Van Look, F. Kakar, et al., "Cesarean Delivery Surveillance System at a Maternity Hospital in Kabul, Afghanistan," *International Journal of Gynaecology & Obstetrics* 104 (2009): 14–17.

64 **she develops a fistula:** See S. Arrowsmith, E. C. Hamlin, and L. L. Wall, "Obstructed Labor Injury Complex: Obstetric Fistula Formation and the Multifaceted Morbidity of Maternal Birth Trauma in the Developing World," *Obstetrical & Gynecological Survey* 51 (1996): 568–74.

64 **Njoki Nganga:** For her story, see Rachel Louise Snyder, "Shunned and Scarred for Life: Can the World's Most Helpless Female Outcasts Be Saved?" *Glamour*, February 2005.

66 **show it to Larry Angel:** Michael J. Weiss, "When the Cops Don't Have a Clue, Larry Angel (a/k/a Sherlock Bones) Makes the Skeletons Talk," *People*, May 16, 1983.

66 **murder victims Angel helped the FBI to identify:** Gretchen A. Grisbaum and Douglas H. Ubelaker, "An Analysis of Forensic Anthropology Cases Submitted to the Smithsonian Institution by the Federal Bureau of Investigation from 1962 to 1994," in *Smithsonian Contributions to Anthropology* (Washington, D.C.: Smithsonian, 2001).

66 **"books just couldn't explain":** Angel is quoted in Michael J. Weiss, "When the Cops Don't Have a Clue, Larry Angel (a/k/a Sherlock Bones) Makes the Skeletons Talk," *People*, May 16, 1983.

66 **measured almost three thousand human skeletons:** J. Lawrence Angel, "Health as a Crucial Factor in the Changes from Hunting to Developed Farming in the Eastern Mediterranean," in *Paleopathology at the Origins of Agriculture*, edited by Mark Nathan Cohen and George J. Armelagos (Orlando: Academic Press, 1984), 51–57.

67 **women now outlive American men:** The difference in life expectancy between men and women has fallen from eight years in the 1970s to five, as predicted from women's increase in cigarette smoking.

67 **the first story:** Stephanie Dalley, *Myths from Mesopotamia* (New York: Oxford University Press, 1991), *Atrahasis* I v, page 25; III vii, page 35.

69 **brain has done much less of its growing when she is born:** The newborn brain of a human is 28 percent the size of the adult brain, while the newborn chimp's is 41 percent of adult size; see Jeremy DeSilva and Julie Lesnik, "Chimpanzee Neonatal Brain Size: Implications for Brain Growth in *Homo erectus*," *Journal of Human Evolution* 51 (2006): 207–12. Also: Harold V. F. Jordaan, "Newborn: Adult Brain Ratios in Hominid Evolution," *American Journal of Physical Anthropology* 44 (1976): 271–78.

69 **why our newborn babies are much fatter:** Stephen C. Cunnane and M. A. Crawford, "Survival of the Fattest: Fat Babies Were the Key to Evolution of the Large Human Brain," *Comparitive Biochemistry and Physiology* 136 A (2003): 17–26. W. D. Bowen, O. T. Oftedal, and D. J. Boness, "Mass and Energy Transfer During Lactation in a Small Phocid, the Harbour Seal (*Phoca vitulina*)," *Physiologic Zoology* 65 (1992): 844–66.

71 **This strong link between a mother's weight:** See, for example: J. A. Kusin, S. Kardjati, and U. H. Renqvist, "Maternal Body Mass Index: The Functional Significance During Reproduction," *European Journal of Clinical Nutrition* 48, suppl. 3 (1994): S56–67; H. A. Abenhaim, R. A. Kinch, L.

Morin, A. Benjamin, R. Usher, Haim A. Abenhaim, Robert A. Kinch, et al., "Effect of Prepregnancy Body Mass Index Categories on Obstetrical and Neonatal Outcomes," *Archives of Gynecology & Obstetrics* 275 (2007): 39–43; L. Ay, C. J. Kruithof, R. Bakker, E. A. Steegers, J. C. Witteman, H. A. Moll, A. Hofman, J. P. Mackenbach, A. C. Hokken-Koelega, et al., "Maternal Anthropometrics Are Associated with Fetal Size in Different Periods of Pregnancy and at Birth," *BJOG: An International Journal of Obstetrics & Gynaecology* 116 (2009): 953–63; A. A. Johnson, E. M. Knight, C. H. Edwards, U. J. Oyemade, O. J. Cole, O. E. Westney, L. S. Westney, H. Laryea, and S. Jones, "Dietary Intakes, Anthropometric Measurements and Pregnancy Outcomes," *Journal of Nutrition* 124 (1994): 936S–942S; Barbara Abrams, S. Carmichael, and S. Selvin, "Factors Associated with the Pattern of Maternal Weight Gain During Pregnancy," *Obstetrics & Gynecology* 86 (1995): 170–76.

71 **Heavier mothers like Marcie tend to eat *less*:** M. M. Bergmann, E. W. Flagg, H. L. Miracle-McMahill, and H. Boeing, "Energy Intake and Net Weight Gain in Pregnant Women According to Body Mass Index (BMI) Status," *International Journal of Obesity* 21 (1997): 1010–7.

71 **more likely to have a baby that is too big:** M. Murakami, M. Ohmichi, T. Takahashi, A. Shibata, A. Fukao, N. Morisaki, and H. Kurachi, "Prepregnancy Body Mass Index as an Important Predictor of Perinatal Outcomes in Japanese," *Archives of Gynecology and Obstetrics* 271 (2005): 311–15.

71 **more likely to have obstructed labor:** G. Barau, P. Y. Robillard, T. C. Hulsey, F. Dedecker, A. Laffite, P. Gerardin, and E. Kauffmann, "Linear Association Between Maternal Pre-Pregnancy Body Mass Index and Risk of Caesarean Section in Term Deliveries," *BJOG: An International Journal of Obstetrics & Gynaecology* 113 (2006): 1173–77. Francis S. Nuthalapaty, Dwight J. Rouse, and John Owen, "The Association of Maternal Weight with Cesarean Risk, Labor Duration, and Cervical Dilation Rate During Labor Induction," *Obstetrics & Gynecology* 103 (2004): 452–56. Sohinee Bhattacharya, Doris M. Campbell, William A. Liston, and Siladitya Bhattacharya, "Effect of Body Mass Index on Pregnancy Outcomes in Nulliparous Women Delivering Singleton Babies," *BMC Public Health* 7 (2007): 168.

72 **waist fat is what mainly determines:** J. E. Brown, J. D. Potter, D. R. Jacobs, Jr., R. A. Kopher, M. J. Rourke, G. M. Barosso, P. J. Hannan, and L. A. Schmid, "Maternal Waist-to-Hip Ratio as a Predictor of Newborn Size," *Epidemiology* 7 (1996): 62–66. Hora Soltani and Robt B. Fraser, "A Longitudinal Study of Maternal Anthropometric Changes in Normal Weight, Overweight and Obese Women During Pregnancy and Postpartum," *British Journal of Nutrition* 84 (2000): 95–101. Elizabeth A. McCarthy, B. J. G. Strauss, S. P. Walker, and M. Permezel, "Determination of Maternal Body Composition in Pregnancy and Its Relevance to Perinatal Outcomes," *Obstetrical & Gynecological Survey* 59 (2004): 731–42. Eliana M. D. R. Wendland, Bruce Bartholow Duncan, Sotero Serrate Mengue, Luciana Bertoldi

Nucci, and Maria Ines Schmidt, "Waist Circumference in the Prediction of Obesity-Related Adverse Pregnancy Outcomes," *Cadernos de Saude Publica* 23 (2007): 391–98.

72 **men will prefer thinner women than they actually do:** George Calden, Richard M. Lundy, and Richard J. Schlafer, "Sex Differences in Body Concepts," *Journal of Consulting Psychology* 23 (1959): 378. Lawrence D. Cohn, Nancy E. Adler, Irwin J. Ce, S. G. Milstein, S. G. Kegeles, and G. Stone, "Body-Figure Preferences in Male and Female Adolescents," *Journal of Abnormal Psychology* 96 (1987): 276–79. April Fallon and Paul Rozin, "Sex Differences in Perceptions of Desirable Body Shape," *Journal of Abnormal Psychology* 94 (1985): 102–5.

73 **super-skinny fashion models:** To make matters worse, images are often doctored to make models appear even thinner. See Ashley Lauren Samsa, "Warning: Models in This Image May Not Be as Thin as They Appear," Ms.Blog (2011), http://msmagazine.com/blog/blog/2011/07/05/warning-models-in-this-image-may-not-be-as-thin-as-they-appear/.

73 **Playmate will still have thirty-two pounds of fat:** This is based on young women in the NHANES sample who match the BMI, height, and waist size of Playmates. Playmates have large amounts of body fat because they are taller than average and have longer legs.

75 **had fat surgically removed:** For statistics on cosmetic fat surgery see www.cosmeticplasticsurgerystatistics.com/statistics.html#2008. Fat removed from the waist is often injected into the hips.

77 **half as many calories:** There are 3,700 calories per person in the American food supply and 2,100 in Bangladesh; men tend to have one and a half times more calories than women. See also D. S. Alam, J. M. A. van Raaij, Jgaj Hautvast, M. Yunus, and G. J. Fuchs, "Energy Stress During Pregnancy and Lactation: Consequences for Maternal Nutrition in Rural Bangladesh," *European Journal of Clinical Nutrition* 57 (2003): 151–56.

77 **Typical of mothers in her country:** This profile is based on data from the World Health Organization and from A. H. Baqui, S. E. Arifeen, S. Amin, and R. E. Black, "Levels and Correlates of Maternal Nutritional Status in Urban Bangladesh," *European Journal of Clinical Nutrition* 48 (1994): 349–57.

77 **lose both weight and fat with each of her pregnancies:** This is called "maternal depletion." See our paper "Changes in Body Fat Distribution in Relation to Parity in American Women: A Covert Form of Maternal Depletion," *American Journal of Physical Anthropology* 131 (2006): 295–302. For Bangladesh, see Sandra L. Huffman, Mark Wolff, and Sarah Lovell, "Nutrition and Fertility in Bangladesh: Nutritional Status of Nonpregnant Women," *American Journal of Clinical Nutrition* 42 (1985): 725–38. A. K. M. Alauddin Chowdhury, "Changes in Maternal Nutritional Status in a Chronically Malnourished Population in Rural Bangladesh," *Ecology of Food and Nutrition* 19 (1987): 201–11.

78 **newborns in Bangladesh:** See D. S. Alam, J. M. A. van Raaij, Jgaj
Hautvast, M. Yunus, and G. J. Fuchs, "Energy Stress During Preg-
nancy and Lactation: Consequences for Maternal Nutrition in Rural
Bangladesh," *European Journal of Clinical Nutrition* 57 (2003): 151–56;
Rubina Shaheen, Andres de Francisco, Shams El Arifeen, Eva-
Charlotte Ekstrom, and Lars Ake Persson, "Effect of Prenatal Food
Supplementation on Birth Weight: An Observational Study from Ban-
gladesh," *American Journal of Clinical Nutrition* 83 (2006): 1355–61.

78 **Susan's ancestral grandmothers:** See Robert William Fogel, *The
Escape from Hunger and Premature Death, 1700–2100.* (Cambridge:
Cambridge University Press, 2004).

79 **researchers at Northwestern University:** Albert W. Hetherington
and Stephen W. Ranson, "Hypothalamic Lesions and Adiposity in
the Rat," *Anatomical Record* 78 (1940): 149–72.

79 **Her hypothalamus:** See J. M. Castellano, J. Roa, R. M. Luque, C.
Dieguez, E. Aguilar, L. Pinilla, and M. Tena-Sempere, "Kiss-1/Kiss-
peptins and the Metabolic Control of Reproduction: Physiologic
Roles and Putative Physiopathological Implications," *Peptides* 30
(2009): 139–45.

80 **enough fat to start having periods:** Velimir Matkovic, J. Z. Ilich,
M. Skugor, N. E. Badenhop, P. Goel, A. Clairmont, D. Klisovic, R.
W. Nahhas, and J. D. Landoll, "Leptin Is Inversely Related to Age at
Menarche in Human Females," *Journal of Clinical Endocrinology and
Metabolism* 82 (1997): 3239–45.

80 **her hypothalamus would have stopped her menstrual cycle:**
See C. K. Welt, J. L. Chan, J. Bullen, R. Murphy, P. Smith, A. M.
DePaoli, A. Karalis, and C. S. Mantzoros, "Recombinant Human
Leptin in Women with Hypothalamic Amenorrhea," *New England
Journal of Medicine* 351 (2004): 987–97.

80 **her hypothalamus allows her to keep:** See Timothy H. Moran,
"Hypothalamic Nutrient Sensing and Energy Balance," *Forum of
Nutrition* 63 (2010): 94–101.

82 **determined by the weight of the woman who receives the egg:**
A. A. Brooks, M. R. Johnson, P. J. Steer, M. E. Pawson, and H. I.
Abdalla, "Birth Weight: Nature or Nurture?" *Early Human Development*
42 (1995): 29–35.

82–83 **tend to have a larger number of children:** Lee Ellis and Dan
Haman, "Population Increases in Obesity Appear to Be Partly Due to
Genetics," *Journal of Biosocial Science* 36 (2004): 547–59. Women
belonging to the Hutterite religious sect averaged more than twelve
children each and were quite well-fed. See Joseph W. Eaton and
Albert J. Mayer, "The Social Biology of Very High Fertility Among
the Hutterites: The Demography of an Unique Population," *Human
Biology* (1953): 206–64.

84 **wants all of a young woman's resources:** Interestingly, polygamous chimp males prefer older females: Martin N. Muller, Melissa Emery Thompson, and Richard W. Wrangham, "Male Chimpanzees Prefer Mating with Old Females," *Current Biology* 16 (2006): 2234–38.

87 **develops a temporary form of diabetes:** See Saju Joy, Niki Istwan, Debbie Rhea, Cheryl Desch, and Gary Stanziano, "The Impact of Maternal Obesity on the Incidence of Adverse Pregnancy Outcomes in High-Risk Term Pregnancies," *American Journal of Perinatology* 26 (2009): 345–49.

87 **serious problems before and after birth:** Nisha Kapoor, Srividhya Sankaran, Steve Hyer, and Hassan Shehata, "Diabetes in Pregnancy: A Review of Current Evidence," *Current Opinion in Obstetrics & Gynecology* 19 (2007): 586–90. Susan Y. Chu, Shin Y. Kim, Joseph Lau, Christopher H. Schmid, Patricia M. Dietz, William M. Callaghan, and Kathryn M. Curtis, "Maternal Obesity and Risk of Stillbirth: A Meta-Analysis," *American Journal of Obstetrics & Gynecology* 197 (2007): 223–28. See also N. A. Beischer, P. Wein, M. T. Sheedy, and B. Steffen, "Identification and Treatment of Women with Hyperglycaemia Diagnosed During Pregnancy Can Significantly Reduce Perinatal Mortality Rates," *Australian & New Zealand Journal of Obstetrics & Gynaecology* 36 (1996): 239–47; T. Cundy, G. Gamble, K. Townend, P. G. Henley, P. MacPherson, and A. B. Roberts, "Perinatal Mortality in Type 2 Diabetes Mellitus," *Diabetic Medicine* 17 (2000): 33–39.

88 **leptin level in her blood:** Leptin is measured in femtograms (10^{-15} grams) per 100 cubic centimeters of blood.

89 **willing for her to take more risks:** The idea that animals take more reproductive risks with age is called the terminal investment hypothesis; see Daniel M. T. Fessler, C. David Navarrete, William Hopkins, and M. Kay Izard, "Examining the Terminal Investment Hypothesis in Humans and Chimpanzees: Associations Among Maternal Age, Parity, and Birth Weight," *American Journal of Physical Anthropology* 127 (2005): 95–104.

96 **brand-new journal article:** Ali H. Mokdad, James S. Marks, Donna F. Stroup, and Julie L. Gerberding, "Actual Causes of Death in the United States, 2000," *Journal of the American Medical Association* 291 (2004): 1238–45.

96 **CBS News:** Bootie Cosgrove-Mather, "Americans Eat Themselves to Death," CBS News, March 9, 2004, www.cbsnews.com/stories/2004/03/09/health/main604956.shtml.

96 ***USA Today*:** Nanci Hellmich, "Obesity on Track as No. 1 Killer," *USA Today*, March 9, 2004.

96 ***Washington Post*:** Rob Stein, "Obesity Passing Smoking as Top Avoidable Cause of Death," *Washington Post*, March 10, 2004.

96 **compared the consequences of the American obesity epidemic:** Jim Kvicala, "Americans Experiencing 'Pandemic of Obesity,' Says Director of Centers for Disease Control and Prevention in Atlanta," in *News at Terry College of Business* (2003), www.terry.uga.edu/news/releases/2003/gerberding.html.

97 **a paper showing that this method:** Katherine M. Flegal, Barry I.
Graubard, and David F. Williamson, "Methods of Calculating Deaths
Attributable to Obesity," *American Journal of Epidemiology* 160 (2004): 331–
38. See also Katherine M. Flegal, David F. Williamson, Elsie R. Pamuk,
and Harry M. Rosenberg, "Estimating Deaths Attributable to Obesity in
the United States," *American Journal of Public Health* 94 (2004): 1486–89.

97 **their own carefully designed study:** Katherine M. Flegal, Barry I.
Graubard, David F. Williamson, and Mitchell H. Gail, "Excess Deaths
Associated with Underweight, Overweight, and Obesity," *Journal of the
American Medical Association* 293 (2005): 1861–67.

97 **health risks of being heavy seemed to be diminishing:** Edward W.
Gregg, Yiling J. Cheng, Betsy L. Cadwell, Giuseppina Imperatore, Des-
mond E. Williams, Katherine M. Flegal, K. M. Venkat Narayan, and
David F. Williamson, "Secular Trends in Cardiovascular Disease Risk
Factors According to Body Mass Index in US Adults," *Journal of the Ameri-
can Medical Association* 293 (2005): 1868–74.

97 **experts in assessing health risks had reviewed her study:** Jennifer
Couzin, "A Heavyweight Battle over CDC's Obesity Forecasts," *Science*
308 (2005): 770–71. See also next note.

97 **thought people would be glad to hear:** Reported in Gina Kolata,
*Rethinking Thin: The New Science of Weight Loss—and the Myths and Realities
of Dieting* (New York: Farrar, Straus & Giroux, 2007), 207.

97 **leading obesity researchers:** See, for example, James O. Hill, "Is
Obesity Bad?" *Obesity Management*, June 2005, 85–86.

98 **commissioned a public opinion poll:** Harvard School of Public
Health press release, "Despite Conflicting Studies About Obesity, Most
Americans Think the Problem Remains Serious," July 14, 2005, www
.hsph.harvard.edu/news/press-releases/archives/2005-releases/
press07142005.html.

98 **Said one:** James O. Hill, "Is Obesity Bad?" *Obesity Management*, June 2005,
85.

98 **She later held a press conference:** Associated Press, "CDC Chief
Backs Away from Report on Obesity," *Washington Post*, June 3, 2005, A07.

98 **David Allison:** D. B. Allison, K. R. Fontaine, J. E. Manson, J. Stevens, and
T. B. VanItallie, "Annual Deaths Attributable to Obesity in the United
States," *Journal of the American Medical Association* 282 (1999): 1530–38.

98 **Selling such products and services:** See Gina Kolata, *Rethinking Thin:
The New Science of Weight Loss—and the Myths and Realities of Dieting* (New
York: Farrar, Straus & Giroux, 2007). Also: W. Wayt Gibbs, "Obesity: An
Overblown Epidemic?" *Scientific American* 292 (2005): 70–77.

99 *women who lose weight live longer:* See T. I. A. Sorensen, "Weight Loss
Causes Increased Mortality: Pros," *Obesity Reviews* 4 (2003): 3–7.

99 **tend to die sooner:** R. Andres, D. C. Muller, and J. D. Sorkin, "Long-
Term Effects of Change in Body Weight on All-Cause Mortality: A
Review," *Annals of Internal Medicine* 119 (1993): 737–43. T. I. A. Sorensen,

"Weight Loss Causes Increased Mortality: Pros," *Obesity Reviews* 4 (2003): 3–7. G. A. Gaesser, "Thinness and Weight Loss: Beneficial or Detrimental to Longevity?" *Medicine & Science in Sports & Exercise* 31 (1999): 1118–28. M. Higgins, R. D'Agostino, W. Kannel, J. Cobb, and J. Pinsky, "Benefits and Adverse Effects of Weight Loss: Observations from the Framingham Study," *Annals of Internal Medicine* 119 (1993): 758–63. Mette K. Simonsen, Yrsa A. Hundrup, Erik B. Obel, Morten Gronbaek, and Berit L. Heitmann, "Intentional Weight Loss and Mortality Among Initially Healthy Men and Women," *Nutrition Reviews* 66 (2008): 375–86.

99   **overweight women like Susan tend to live longer:** Daniel L. McGee, "Body Mass Index and Mortality: A Meta-Analysis Based on Person-Level Data from Twenty-six Observational Studies," *Annals of Epidemiology* 15 (2005): 87–97. Soham Al Snih, Kenneth J. Ottenbacher, Kyriakos S. Markides, Yong-Fang Kuo, Karl Eschbach, and James S. Goodwin, "The Effect of Obesity on Disability vs. Mortality in Older Americans," *Archives of Internal Medicine* 167 (2007): 774–80. Ramon A. Durazo-Arvizu, D. L. McGee, R. S. Cooper, Y. Liao, and A. Luke, "Mortality and Optimal Body Mass Index in a Sample of the US Population," *American Journal of Clinical Nutrition* 147 (1998): 739–49. Leon Flicker, Kieran A. McCaul, Graeme J. Hankey, Konrad Jamrozik, Wendy J. Brown, Julie E. Byles, and Osvaldo P. Almeida, "Body Mass Index and Survival in Men and Women Aged 70 to 75," *Journal of the American Geriatrics Society* 58 (2010): 234–41. S. W. Farrell, L. Braun, C. E. Barlow, Y. J. Cheng, and S. N. Blair, "The Relation of Body Mass Index, Cardiorespiratory Fitness, and All-Cause Mortality in Women," *Obesity Research* 10 (2002): 417–23. Ian Janssen, "Morbidity and Mortality Risk Associated with an Overweight BMI in Older Men and Women," *Obesity* 15 (2007): 1827–40. Esa Laara and P. Rantakallio, "Body Size and Mortality in Women: A 29 Year Follow-Up of 12,000 Pregnant Women in Northern Finland," *Journal of Epidemiology and Community Health* 50 (1996): 408–14. Paula M. Lantz, Ezra Golberstein, James S. House, and Jeffrey Morenoff, "Socioeconomic and Behavioral Risk Factors for Mortality in a National 19-Year Prospective Study of U.S. Adults," *Social Science & Medicine* 70 (2010): 1558–66. K. G. Losonczy, T. B. Harris, J. Cornoni-Huntley, E. M. Simonsick, R. B. Wallace, N. R. Cook, A. M. Ostfeld, and D. G. Blazer, "Does Weight Loss from Middle Age to Old Age Explain the Inverse Weight Mortality Relation in Old Age?" *American Journal of Epidemiology* 141 (1995): 312–21. J. E. Manson, W. C. Willett, M. J. Stampfer, G. A. Colditz, D. J. Hunter, S. E. Hankinson, C. H. Hennekens, and F. E. Speizer, "Body Weight and Mortality Among Women," *New England Journal of Medicine* 333 (1995): 677–85. H. M. Orpana, J. M. Berthelot, M. S. Kaplan, D. H. Feeny, B. McFarland, and N. A. Ross, "BMI and Mortality: Results from a National Longitudinal Study of Canadian Adults," *Obesity* 18 (2010): 214–18. June Stevens, Junwen Cai, Juhaeri, Michael J. Thun, David F. Williamson, and Joy L. Wood,

"Consequences of the Use of Different Measures of Effect to Determine the Impact of Age on the Association Between Obesity and Mortality," *American Journal of Epidemiology* 150 (1999): 399–407. X. Sui, M. J. LaMonte, J. N. Laditka, J. W. Hardin, N. Chase, S. P. Hooker, et al., "Cardiorespiratory Fitness and Adiposity as Mortality Predictors in Older Adults," *Journal of the American Medical Association* 298 (2007): 2507–16. Hans T. Waaler, "Height, Weight and Mortality: The Norwegian Experience," *Acta Medica Scandinavica* 215, suppl. 679 (1984): 1–56. P. E. Wändell, A. C. Carlsson, and H. Theobald, "The Association Between BMI Value and Long-Term Mortality," *International Journal of Obesity* 33 (2009): 577–82. S. Zhu, M. Heo, M. Plankey, M. S. Faith, and D. B. Allison, "Associations of Body Mass Index and Anthropometric Indicators of Fat Mass and Fat Free Mass with All-Cause Mortality Among Women in the First and Second National Health and Nutrition Examination Surveys," *Annals of Epidemiology* 13 (2003): 286–93. Matthias Lenz, Tanja Richter, and Ingrid Muhlhauser, "The Morbidity and Mortality Associated with Overweight and Obesity in Adulthood: A Systematic Review," *Deutsches Arzteblatt International* 106 (2009): 641–48.

99 **problems with their methods:** Most studies showing increased mortality in overweight are based on self-reported weights, which overestimate effects of BMI: see A. Chiolero, I. Peytremann-Bridevaux, and F. Paccaud, "Associations between Obesity and Health Conditions May Be Overestimated If Self-Reported Body Mass Index Is Used," *Obesity Reviews* 8 (2007): 373–74.

99 **some studies show a small decrease in life span:** Ramon A. Durazo-Arvizu, D. L. McGee, R. S. Cooper, Y. Liao, and A. Luke, "Mortality and Optimal Body Mass Index in a Sample of the US Population," *American Journal of Clinical Nutrition* 147 (1998): 739–49. M. G. Jain, A. B. Miller, T. E. Rohan, J. T. Rehm, S. J. Bondy, M. J. Ashley, J. E. Cohen, and R. G. Ferrence, "Body Mass Index and Mortality in Women: Follow-Up of the Canadian National Breast Screening Study Cohort," *International Journal of Obesity* 29 (2005): 792–97. P. T. Katzmarzyk, C. L. Craig, and C. Bouchard, "Underweight, Overweight and Obesity: Relationships with Mortality in the 13-Year Follow-Up of the Canada Fitness Survey," *Journal of Clinical Epidemiology* 54 (2001): 916–20. Prospective Studies Collaboration, "Body-Mass Index and Cause-Specific Mortality in 900,000 Adults: Collaborative Analyses of 57 Prospective Studies," *Lancet* 373 (2009): 1083–96.

99 **many show no survival difference:** Julie A. Simpson, Robert J. MacInnis, Anna Peeters, John L. Hopper, Graham G. Giles, and Dallas R. English, "A Comparison of Adiposity Measures as Predictors of All-Cause Mortality: The Melbourne Collaborative Cohort Study," *Obesity* 15 (2007): 994–1003. J. C. Seidell, W. M. Verschuren, E. M. van Leer, and D. Kromhout, "Overweight, Underweight, and Mortality: A Prospective

Study of 48,287 Men and Women," *Archives of Internal Medicine* 156 (1996): 958–63. T. L. Visscher, J. C. Seidell, A. Molarius, D. van der Kuip, A. Hofman, and J. C. Witteman, "A Comparison of Body Mass Index, Waist-Hip Ratio and Waist Circumference as Predictors of All-Cause Mortality Among the Elderly: The Rotterdam Study," *International Journal of Obesity* 25 (2001): 1730–35. T. A. Welborn, M. W. Knuiman, and H. T. Vu, "Body Mass Index and Alternative Indices of Obesity in Relation to Height, Triceps Skinfold and Subsequent Mortality: The Busselton Health Study," *International Journal of Obesity* 24 (2000): 108–15. J. Klenk, G. Nagel, H. Ulmer, A. Strasak, H. Concin, G. Diem, K., et al. , "Body Mass Index and Mortality: Results of a Cohort of 184,697 Adults in Austria," *European Journal of Epidemiology* 24 (2009): 83–91. L. Iversen, P. C. Hannaford, A. J. Lee, A. M. Elliott, S. Fielding, Lisa Iversen, Philip C. Hannaford, Amanda J. Lee, Alison M. Elliott, and Shona Fielding, "Impact of Lifestyle in Middle-Aged Women on Mortality: Evidence from the Royal College of General Practitioners' Oral Contraception Study," *British Journal of General Practice* 60 (2010): 563–69. Masato Nagai, Shinichi Kuriyama, Masako Kakizaki, Kaori Ohmori-Matsuda, Yumi Sugawara, Toshimasa Sone, Atsushi Hozawa, and Ichiro Tsuji, "Effect of Age on the Association Between Body Mass Index and All-Cause Mortality: The Ohsaki Cohort Study," *Journal of Epidemiology* 20 (2010): 398–407.

99 **survival is highest in this group:** Fulvia Seccareccia, M. Lanti, A. Menotti, and M. Scanga, "Role of Body Mass Index in the Prediction of All Cause Mortality in over 62,000 Men and Women: The Italian Rifle Pooling Project," *Journal of Epidemiology and Community Health* 52 (1998): 20–26. K. R. Fontaine, M. Heo, L. J. Cheskin, and D. B. Allison, "Body Mass Index, Smoking, and Mortality Among Older American Women," *Journal of Women's Health* 7 (1998): 1257–61. D. B. Allison, D. Gallagher, M. Heo, F. X. Pi-Sunyer, and S. B. Heymsfield, "Body Mass Index and All-Cause Mortality Among People Age 70 and Over: The Longitudinal Study of Aging," *International Journal of Obesity* 21 (1997): 424–31. Soham Al Snih, Kenneth J. Ottenbacher, Kyriakos S. Markides, Yong-Fang Kuo, Karl Eschbach, and James S. Goodwin, "The Effect of Obesity on Disability vs. Mortality in Older Americans," *Archives of Internal Medicine* 167 (2007): 774–80. A. M. Beck and K. Damkjaer, "Optimal Body Mass Index in a Nursing Home Population," *Journal of Nutritional Health and Aging* 12 (2008): 675–77. G. M. Price, R. Uauy, E. Breeze, C. J. Bulpitt, and A. E. Fletcher, "Weight, Shape, and Mortality Risk in Older Persons: Elevated Waist-Hip Ratio, Not High Body Mass Index, Is Associated with a Greater Risk of Death," *American Journal of Clinical Nutrition* 84 (2006): 449–60. Avraham Weiss, Yichayaou Beloosesky, Mona Boaz, Alexandra Yalov, Ran Kornowski, and Ehud Grossman, "Body Mass Index Is Inversely Related to Mortality in Elderly Subjects," *Journal of General Internal Medicine* 23 (2008): 19–24.

99   **a loss of about eight years is typical:** Prospective Studies Collaboration, "Body-Mass Index and Cause-Specific Mortality in 900 000 Adults: Collaborative Analyses of 57 Prospective Studies," *Lancet* 373 (2009): 1083–96.

99   **Obese women who are physically active have much better survival:** Frank B. Hu, Walter C. Willett, Tricia Li, Meir J. Stampfer, Graham A. Colditz, and JoAnn E. Manson, "Adiposity as Compared with Physical Activity in Predicting Mortality Among Women," *New England Journal of Medicine* 351 (2004): 2694–2703. Annemarie Koster, Tamara B. Harris, Steven C. Moore, Arthur Schatzkin, Albert R. Hollenbeck, Jacques Th. M. van Eijk, and Michael F. Leitzmann, "Joint Associations of Adiposity and Physical Activity with Mortality: The National Institutes of Health-AARP Diet and Health Study," *American Journal of Epidemiology* 169 (2009): 1344–51. Xuemei Sui, Michael J. LaMonte, James N. Laditka, James W. Hardin, Nancy Chase, Steven P. Hooker, and Steven N. Blair, "Cardiorespiratory Fitness and Adiposity as Mortality Predictors in Older Adults," *Journal of the American Medical Association* 298 (2007): 2507–16. Deborah Riebe, Bryan J. Blissmer, Mary L. Greaney, Carol Ewing Garber, Faith D. Lees, and Philip G. Clark, "The Relationship Between Obesity, Physical Activity, and Physical Function in Older Adults," *Journal of Aging & Health* 21 (2009): 1159–78. M. Fogelholm, "Physical Activity, Fitness and Fatness: Relations to Mortality, Morbidity and Disease Risk Factors: A Systematic Review," *Obesity Reviews* 11 (2010): 202–21.

100   **other adverse health effects unconnected with weight:** Genes related to obesity include genes involved with growth, metabolism, and immune and neuronal processes: E. K. Speliotes, C. J. Willer, S. I. Berndt, K. L. Monda, G. Thorleifsson, A. U. Jackson, H. L. Allen, C. M. Lindgren, J. Luan, R. Magi, et al., "Association Analyses of 249,796 Individuals Reveal 18 New Loci Associated with Body Mass Index," *Nature Genetics* 42 (2010): 937–48.

100   **good for the health of all women:** B. M. Yashodhara, S. Umakanth, J. M. Pappachan, S. K. Bhat, R. Kamath, and B. H. Choo, "Omega-3 Fatty Acids: A Comprehensive Review of Their Role in Health and Disease," *Postgraduate Medical Journal* 85 (2009): 84–90. N. D. Riediger, R. A. Othman, M. Suh, and M. H. Moghadasian, "A Systemic Review of the Roles of N-3 Fatty Acids in Health and Disease," *Journal of the American Dietetic Association* 109 (2009): 668–79. Philip C. Calder and Parveen Yaqoob, "Omega-3 Polyunsaturated Fatty Acids and Human Health Outcomes," *Biofactors* 35 (2009): 266–72. Artemis P. Simopoulos, "The Importance of the Omega-6/Omega-3 Fatty Acid Ratio in Cardiovascular Disease and Other Chronic Diseases," *Experimental Biology & Medicine* 233 (2008): 674–88.

101   **to get or die from tuberculosis:** A. Tverdal, "Body Mass Index and Incidence of Tuberculosis," *European Journal of Respiratory Diseases* 69 (1986): 355–62. C. C. Leung, T. H. Lam, W. M. Chan, W. W. Yew, K. S.

Ho, G. Leung, W. S. Law, C. M. Tam, et al., "Lower Risk of Tuberculosis in Obesity," *Archives of Internal Medicine* 167 (2007): 1297–1304. Hans T. Waaler, "Height, Weight and Mortality: The Norwegian Experience," *Acta Medica Scandinavica*, suppl. 679 (1984): 1–56.

101 **lower weights are the most likely to die from infections:** M. E. Falagas, A. P. Athanasoulia, G. Peppas, and D. E. Karageorgopoulos, "Effect of Body Mass Index on the Outcome of Infections: A Systematic Review," *Obesity Reviews* 10 (2009): 280–89.

102 **death rate from infections is one-third lower:** See our paper "Costs and Benefits of Fat-Free Muscle Mass in Men: Relationship to Mating Success, Dietary Requirements, and Native Immunity," *Evolution and Human Behavior* 30 (2009): 322–28.

103 **estrogen blocks their effects on her blood vessels:** G. A. Colditz, W. C. Willett, M. J. Stampfer, B. Rosner, F. E. Speizer, and C. H. Hennekens, "Menopause and the Risk of Coronary Heart Disease in Women," *New England Journal of Medicine* 316 (1987): 1105–10.

103 **many young American soldiers:** William F. Enos, Robert H. Holmes, and James Beyer, "Coronary Disease Among United States Soldiers Killed in Action in Korea: Preliminary Report," *Journal of the American Medical Association* 152 (1953): 1090–93.

103 **women have been *seven times* less likely than men to die of coronary disease:** See, for example, "Variations in Mortality from Coronary Disease," *Statistical Bulletin* 38 June (1957): 1–3.

103 **smoking cuts this benefit in half:** E. Prescott, H. Scharling, M. Osler, and P. Schnohr, "Importance of Light Smoking and Inhalation Habits on Risk of Myocardial Infarction and All Cause Mortality: A 22-Year Follow-Up of 12,149 Men and Women in the Copenhagen City Heart Study," *Journal of Epidemiology and Community Health* 56 (2002): 702–6.

103 **convert more of their natural testosterone to estrogen:** N. I. Williams, J. L. Reed, H. J. Leidy, R. S. Legro, and M. J. De Souza, "Estrogen and Progesterone Exposure Is Reduced in Response to Energy Deficiency in Women Aged 25–40 Years," *Human Reproduction* 25 (2010): 2328–39.

104 **heavier in their teens have *less* chance of developing breast cancer:** Heather J. Baer, Shelley S. Tworoger, Susan E. Hankinson, and Walter C. Willett, "Body Fatness at Young Ages and Risk of Breast Cancer Throughout Life," *American Journal of Epidemiology* 171 (2010): 1183–94.

104 **one in nine American women develop breast cancer:** This is based on statistics from the National Cancer Institute, available at www.cancer .gov/cancertopics/factsheet/detection/probability-breast-cancer.

104 **breast cancer after fifty increases by a fourth:** P. A. van den Brandt, D. Spiegelman, S. S. Yaun, H. O. Adami, L. Beeson, A. R. Folsom, et al., "Pooled Analysis of Prospective Cohort Studies on Height, Weight, and Breast Cancer Risk," *American Journal of Epidemiology* 152 (2000): 514–27.

See also: http://seer.cancer.gov/csr/1975_2007/results_merged/topic _lifetime_risk.pdf.

104 **omega-3 fats reduce the chances of breast cancer:** A. C. Thiebaut, V. Chajes, M. Gerber, M. C. Boutron-Ruault, V. Joulin, G. Lenoir, F. Berrino, E. Riboli, J. Benichou, and F. Clavel-Chapelon, "Dietary Intakes of Omega-6 and Omega-3 Polyunsaturated Fatty Acids and the Risk of Breast Cancer," *International Journal of Cancer* 124 (2009): 924–31. M. Gago-Dominguez, J. M. Yuan, C. L. Sun, H. P. Lee, and M. C. Yu, "Opposing Effects of Dietary N-3 and N-6 Fatty Acids on Mammary Carcinogenesis: The Singapore Chinese Health Study," *British Journal of Cancer* 89 (2003): 1686–92.

105 **high-omega-3/low-omega-6 diet can also help to prevent diabetes:** Dawn Fedor and Darshan S. Kelley, "Prevention of Insulin Resistance by n-3 Polyunsaturated Fatty Acids," *Current Opinion in Clinical Nutrition & Metabolic Care* 12 (2009): 138–46.

105 **Women with the highest weights have just one-third the hip-fracture risk:** Emily D. Parker, Mark A. Pereira, Beth Virnig, and Aaron R. Folsom, "The Association of Hip Circumference with Incident Hip Fracture in a Cohort of Postmenopausal Women," *Annals of Epidemiology* 18 (2008): 836–41.

105 **kind of compensation:** R. G. Cumming and R. J. Klineberg, "Epidemiological Study of the Relation Between Arthritis of the Hip and Hip Fractures," *Annals of the Rheumatic Diseases* 52 (1993): 707–10.

106 ***not* losing weight and having strong bones:** R. S. Newson, J. C. Witteman, O. H. Franco, B. H. Stricker, M. M. Breteler, A. Hofman, and H. Tiemeier, "Predicting Survival and Morbidity-Free Survival to Very Old Age," *Age* 32 (2010): 521–34.

106 **waist size is more important than weight alone:** H. J. Schneider, N. Friedrich, J. Klotsche, L. Pieper, M. Nauck, U. John, et al., "The Predictive Value of Different Measures of Obesity for Incident Cardiovascular Events and Mortality," *Journal of Clinical Endocrinology & Metabolism* 95 (2010): 1777–85. P. K. Myint, A. A. Welch, R. N. Luben, N. W. Wainwright, P. G. Surtees, S. A. Bingham, N. J. Wareham, R. D. Smith, I. M. Harvey, and K. T. Khaw, "Obesity Indices and Self-Reported Functional Health in Men and Women in the Epic-Norfolk," *Obesity* 14 (2006): 884–93.

106 **tend to have less health-promoting omega-3:** Maria Garaulet, F. Perez-Llamas, M. Perez-Ayala, P. Martinez, F. S. de Medina, F. J. Tebar, and S. Zamora, "Site-Specific Differences in the Fatty Acid Composition of Abdominal Adipose Tissue in an Obese Population from a Mediterranean Area," *American Journal of Clinical Nutrition* 74 (2001): 585–91. Shun Wang, Aiqun Ma, Shaowu Song, Qinghai Quan, Xinfeng Zhao, and Xiaohui Zheng, "Fasting Serum Free Fatty Acid Composition, Waist/Hip

Ratio and Insulin Activity in Essential Hypertensive Patients," *Hypertension Research* 31 (2008): 623–32.

106 **those with more lower-body fat:** Peter Lindqvist, Kate Andersson, Valter Sundh, Lauren Lissner, Cecilia Bjorkelund, and Calle Bengtsson, "Concurrent and Separate Effects of Body Mass Index and Waist-to-Hip Ratio on 24-Year Mortality in the Population Study of Women in Gothenburg," *European Journal of Epidemiology* 21 (2006): 789–94. Lauren Lissner, Cecilia Bjorkelund, L. Berit, Jaap C. Heitmann, and Calle Bengtsson Seidell, "Larger Hip Circumference Independently Predicts Health and Longevity in a Swedish Female Cohort," *Obesity Research* 9 (2001): 644–46. C. Mason, C. L. Craig, P. T. Katzmarzyk, Caitlin Mason, Cora L. Craig, and Peter T. Katzmarzyk, "Influence of Central and Extremity Circumferences on All-Cause Mortality in Men and Women," *Obesity* 16 (2008): 2690–95. Preethi Srikanthan, Teresa E. Seeman, and Arun S. Karlamangla, "Waist-Hip Ratio as a Predictor of All-Cause Mortality in High-Functioning Older Adults," *Annals of Epidemiology* 19 (2009): 724–31. Cuilin Zhang, Kathryn M. Rexrode, Rob M. van Dam, Tricia Y. Li, and Frank B. Hu, "Abdominal Obesity and the Risk of All-Cause, Cardiovascular, and Cancer Mortality: Sixteen Years of Follow-Up in US Women," *Circulation* 117 (2008): 1658–67. C. D. Pengelly, and J. Morris, "Body Mass Index and Weight Distribution," *Scottish Medical Journal* 54 (2009): 17–21.

106 **waist size over thirty-five inches:** Ian Janssen, P. T. Katzmarzyk, and R. Ross, "Body Mass Index, Waist Circumference, and Health Risk," *Archives of Internal Medicine* 162 (2002): 2074–79. Petra H. Lahmann, L. Lissner, B. Gullberg, and G. Berglund, "A Prospective Study of Adiposity and All-Cause Mortality: The Malmo Diet and Cancer Study," *Obesity Research* 10 (2002): 361–69. Julie A. Simpson, Robert J. MacInnis, Anna Peeters, John L. Hopper, Graham G. Giles, and Dallas R. English, "A Comparison of Adiposity Measures as Predictors of All-Cause Mortality: The Melbourne Collaborative Cohort Study," *Obesity* 15 (2007): 994–1003. See also www.nhlbi.nih.gov/health/public/heart/obesity/lose_wt/risk.htm.

107 **poorer health later in life:** Rob M. van Dam, W. C. Willett, J. E. Manson, and F. B. Hu, "The Relationship Between Overweight in Adolescence and Premature Death in Women," *Annals of Internal Medicine* 145 (2006): 91–92. Eric N. Reither, Robert M. Hauser, and Karen C. Swallen, "Predicting Adult Health and Mortality from Adolescent Facial Characteristics in Yearbook Photographs," *Demography* 46 (2009): 27–41. Anders Engeland, T. Bjorge, A. J. Sogaard, and A. Tverdal, "Body Mass Index in Adolescence in Relation to Total Mortality: 32-Year Follow-Up in 227,000 Boys and Girls," *American Journal of Epidemiology* 157 (2003): 51723.

107 **three out of four developed diabetes:** K. M. Narayan, J. P. Boyle, T. J. Thompson, E. W. Gregg, and D. F. Williamson, "Effect of BMI on Lifetime Risk for Diabetes in the U.S.," *Diabetes Care* 30 (2007): 1562–66.

Paul W. Franks, Robert L. Hanson, William C. Knowler, Maurice L. Sievers, Peter H. Bennett, and Helen C. Looker, "Childhood Obesity, Other Cardiovascular Risk Factors, and Premature Death," *New England Journal of Medicine* 362 (2010): 485–93.

107 **heavier women are healthier today:** Edward W. Gregg, Yiling J. Cheng, Betsy L. Cadwell, Giuseppina Imperatore, Desmond E. Williams, Katherine M. Flegal, K. M. Venkat Narayan, and David F. Williamson, "Secular Trends in Cardiovascular Disease Risk Factors according to Body Mass Index in US Adults," *Journal of the American Medical Association* 293 (2005): 1868–74. Katherine M. Flegal, Barry I. Graubard, David F. Williamson, and Mitchell H. Gail, "Excess Deaths Associated with Underweight, Overweight, and Obesity," *Journal of the American Medical Association* 293 (2005): 1861–67. Kenneth G. Manton, XiLiang Gu, and Gene R. Lowrimore, "Cohort Changes in Active Life Expectancy in the U.S. Elderly Population: Experience from the 1982–2004 National Long-Term Care Survey," *Journals of Gerontology Series B—Psychological Sciences & Social Sciences* 63 (2008): S269–81.

110 **thirty-six conscientious objectors:** Jeffrey is a composite drawn from data and descriptions of volunteer behavior in Ancel Keys, J. Brozek, A. Henschel, O. Mickelsen, and H. L. Taylor, *The Biology of Human Starvation* (Minneapolis: University of Minnesotta Press, 1950).

111 **Jules Hirsch:** M. L. Glucksman and J. Hirsch, "The Response of Obese Patients to Weight Reduction: A Clinical Evaluation of Behavior," *Psychosomatic Medicine* 30 (1968): 1–11. Jules Hirsch, "The Search for New Ways to Treat Obesity," *Proceedings of the National Academy of Sciences* 99 (2002): 9096–97.

112 **Ethan Sims:** Sims's experiments with mice are discussed by Gina Kolata in *Rethinking Thin: The New Science of Weight Loss—and the Myths and Realities of Dieting* (New York: Farrar, Straus & Giroux, 2007). The experience of Winston Morris is from Ethan A. H. Sims and Edward S. Horton, "Endocrine and Metabolic Adaptation to Obesity and Starvation," *American Journal of Clinical Nutrition* 21 (1968): 1455–79.

112 **Gina Kolata:** *Rethinking Thin: The New Science of Weight Loss—and the Myths and Realities of Dieting* (New York: Farrar, Straus & Giroux, 2007).

113 **Jim Lewis and Jim Springer:** These twins were part of the Minnesota Twin Study and are described in Nancy Segal's book *Entwined Lives: Twins and What They Tell Us About Human Behavior* (New York: Dutton, 1999).

113–14 **two-thirds of the differences in weight:** Albert J. Stunkard, Jennifer R. Harris, Nancy L Pedersen, and George E. McClearn, "The Body-Mass Index of Twins Who Have Been Reared Apart," *New England Journal of Medicine* 322 (1990): 1483–87. M. Korkeila, J.

Kaprio, A. Rissanen, and M. Koskenvuo, "Consistency and Change of Body Mass Index and Weight: A Study on 5967 Adult Finnish Twin Pairs," *International Journal of Obesity* 19 (1995): 310–17.

114 **the average was 117 pounds:** Low weights after 18 come from the NHANES I 1971–75. The weights in this paragraph are derived from BMIs adjusted for an average height of sixty-four inches.

114 **same question about their low weight at eighteen:** The question was asked again in the NHANES 1999–2000.

115 **more frequently women diet, the more they gain:** Juhaeri, J. Steven, L. E. Chambless, H. A. Tyroler, J. Harp, D. Jones, and D. Arnett, "Weight Change Among Self-Reported Dieters and Non-Dieters in White and African American Men and Women," *European Journal of Epidemiology* 17 (2001): 917–23. A. Kroke, A. D. Liese, M. Schulz, M. M. Bergmann, K. Klipstein-Grobusch, K. Hoffmann, and H. Boeing, "Recent Weight Changes and Weight Cycling as Predictors of Subsequent Two Year Weight Change in a Middle-Aged Cohort," *International Journal of Obesity* 26 (2002): 403–9. Jennifer S. Savage, Lesa Hoffman, and Leann L. Birch, "Dieting, Restraint, and Disinhibition Predict Women's Weight Change over 6 Y," *American Journal of Clinical Nutrition* 90 (2009): 33–40. E. Stice, R. P. Cameron, J. D. Killen, C. Hayward, and C. B. Taylor, "Naturalistic Weight-Reduction Efforts Prospectively Predict Growth in Relative Weight and Onset of Obesity Among Female Adolescents," *Journal of Consulting & Clinical Psychology* 67 (1999): 967–74. Gretchen Van Wye, Joel A. Dubin, Steven N. Blair, and Loretta Di Pietro, "Weight Cycling and 6-Year Weight Change in Healthy Adults," *Obesity* 15 (2007): 731–39. Wronique Provencher, Vicky Drapeau, Angelo Tremblay, Jean-Pierre Despres, Claude Bouchard, and Simone Lemieux, "Eating Behaviours, Dietary Profile and Body Composition According to Dieting History in Men and Women of the Quebec Family Study," *British Journal of Nutrition* 91 (2004): 997–1004.

115 **a group of overweight nurses:** A. E. Field, J. E. Manson, C. B. Taylor, W. C. Willett, and G. A. Colditz, "Association of Weight Change, Weight Control Practices, and Weight Cycling among Women in the Nurses' Health Study II," *International Journal of Obesity* 28 (2004): 1134–42.

117 **more likely to have their babies when food supplies are high:** S. Becker, "Seasonality of Fertility in Matlab, Bangladesh," *Journal of Biosocial Science* 13 (1981): 97–106.

117 **more likely to give birth during the harvest season:** According to U.S. natality data for all births in 2005, there were 20 percent more babies born in August than in February, and 32 percent more in Nevada.

118–19 **fat cells become more and more reluctant:** Simon Schenk, Matthew P. Harber, Cara R. Shrivastava, Charles F. Burant, and Jeffrey F. Horowitz, "Improved Insulin Sensitivity After Weight Loss and Exercise Training Is Mediated by a Reduction in Plasma Fatty Acid Mobilization, Not Enhanced Oxidative Capacity," *Journal of Physiology* 587 (2009): 4949–61.

120 **reward centers light up for high-calorie foods:** A. P. Goldstone, C. G. de Hernandez, J. D. Beaver, K. Muhammed, C. Croese, G. Bell, G. Durighel, E. Hughes, et al., "Fasting Biases Brain Reward Systems toward High-Calorie Foods," *European Journal of Neuroscience* 30 (2009): 1625–35.

120 **higher levels of the hormones that increase her appetite:** L. E. Hooper, K. E. Foster-Schubert, D. S. Weigle, B. Sorensen, C. M. Ulrich, and A. McTiernan, "Frequent Intentional Weight Loss Is Associated with Higher Ghrelin and Lower Glucose and Androgen Levels in Postmenopausal Women," *Nutrition Research* 30 (2010): 163–70.

120 **store more of her calories as fat:** Z. Kochan, J. Karbowska, and J. Swierczynski, "The Effects of Weight Cycling on Serum Leptin Levels and Lipogenic Enzyme Activities in Adipose Tissue," *Journal of Physiology & Pharmacology* 57, suppl. 6 (2006): 115–27.

120 **burn less of it:** F. Froidevaux, Y. Schutz, L. Christin, and E. Jequier, "Energy Expenditure in Obese Women Before and During Weight Loss, after Refeeding, and in the Weight-Relapse Period," *American Journal of Clinical Nutrition* 57 (1993): 35–42.

120 **have a slower metabolism:** Irene Strychar, Marie-Eve Lavoie, Lyne Messier, Antony D. Karelis, Eric Doucet, et al., "Anthropometric, Metabolic, Psychosocial, and Dietary Characteristics of Overweight/ Obese Postmenopausal Women with a History of Weight Cycling," *Journal of the American Dietetic Association* 109 (2009): 718–24.

120 **more inclined to hold on to fat:** Barbara A. Gower, Gary R. Hunter, Paula C. Chandler-Laney, Jessica A. Alvarez, and Nikki C. Bush, "Glucose Metabolism and Diet Predict Changes in Adiposity and Fat Distribution in Weight-Reduced Women," *Obesity* 18 (2010): 1532–37.

120 **a study of a group of obese Italian women:** Z. L. Benini, M. A. Camilloni, C. Scordato, G. Lezzi, G. Savia, G. Oriani, S. Bertoli, F. Balzola, A. Liuzzi, and M. L. Petroni, "Contribution of Weight Cycling to Serum Leptin in Human Obesity," *International Journal of Obesity* 25 (2001): 721–26.

120 **increase blood pressure:** M. Schulz, A. D. Liese, H. Boeing, J. E. Cunningham, C. G. Moore, and A. Kroke, "Associations of Short-Term Weight Changes and Weight Cycling with Incidence of Essential Hypertension in the Epic-Potsdam Study," *Journal of Human Hypertension* 19 (2005): 61–67.

120 **decrease good cholesterol:** M. B. Olson, S. F. Kelsey, V. Bittner, S. E. Reis, N. Reichek, E. M. Handberg, and C. N. Merz, "Weight Cycling and High-Density Lipoprotein Cholesterol in Women: Evidence of an Adverse Effect," *Journal of the American College of Cardiology* 36 (2000): 1565–71.

120 **increase inflammation:** K. Strohacker and B. K. McFarlin, "Influence of Obesity, Physical Inactivity, and Weight Cycling on Chronic Inflammation," *Frontiers in Bioscience* 2 (2010): 98–104.

120 **reduce life span:** K. D. Brownell and J. Rodin, "Medical, Metabolic, and Psychological Effects of Weight Cycling," *Archives of Internal Medicine* 154 (1994): 1325–30. M. W. Reynolds, L. Fredman, P. Langenberg, and J. Magaziner, "Weight, Weight Change, Mortality in a Random Sample of Older Community-Dwelling Women," *Journal of the American Geriatrics Society* 47 (1999): 1409–14. E. Muls, K. Kempen, G. Vansant, and W. Saris, "Is Weight Cycling Detrimental to Health? A Review of the Literature in Humans," *International Journal of Obesity* 19, suppl. 3 (1995): S46–50.

120 **added waist fat:** J. Rodin, N. Radke-Sharpe, M. Rebuffe-Scrive, and M. R. Greenwood, "Weight Cycling and Fat Distribution," *International Journal of Obesity* 14 (1990): 303–10. S. J. Wallner, N. Luschnigg, W. J. Schnedl, T. Lahousen, K. Sudi, K. Crailsheim, R. Moller, E. Tafeit, and R. Horejsi, "Body Fat Distribution of Overweight Females with a History of Weight Cycling," *International Journal of Obesity* 28 (2004): 1143–48.

120 **more likely to be depressed:** J. P. Foreyt, R. L. Brunner, G. K. Goodrick, G. Cutter, K. D. Brownell, and S. T. St. Jeor, "Psychological Correlates of Weight Fluctuation," *International Journal of Eating Disorders* 17 (1995): 263–75.

120 **decrease in mental ability:** P. J. Rogers and M. W. Green, "Dieting, Dietary Restraint and Cognitive Performance," *British Journal of Clinical Psychology* 32 (1993): 113–16.

121 **a woman in the weight-loss study discussed by Gina Kolata:** Gina Kolata, *Rethinking Thin* (New York: Farrar, Straus & Giroux, 2007), 216.

123 **this has been shown in animals:** Vincenzo Di Marzo and Isabel Matias, "Endocannabinoid Control of Food Intake and Energy Balance," *Nature Neuroscience* 8 (2005): 585–89.

126 **its good fats are overwhelmed and blocked:** See H. Chung, J. A. Nettleton, R. N. Lemaitre, R. G. Barr, M. Y. Tsai, R. P. Tracy, and D. S. Siscovick, "Frequency and Type of Seafood Consumed Influence Plasma (N-3) Fatty Acid Concentrations," *Journal of Nutrition* 138 (2008): 2422–27.

128 **at least 250 milligrams a day of DHA:** American Heart Assocation: www.heart.org/idc/groups/heart-public/@wcm/@adv/documents /downloadable/ucm_312853.pdf. Artemis P. Simopoulos, L. Leaf, and N. Salem, Jr., "Workshop on the Essentiality of and Recommended Dietary Intakes for Omega-6 and Omega-3 Fatty Acids," *Journal of the American College of Nutrition* 18 (1999): 487–89. International Society for

the Study of Fatty Acids and Lipids: www.issfal.org/index.php?option=
com_content&task=view&id=23&Itemid=8.

128 **some experts recommend more than four times as much:** Some
recommend 1.7 grams of DHA and EPA for those with an American diet:
Joseph R. Hibbeln, Levi R. G. Nieminen, Tanya L. Blasbalg, Jessica A.
Riggs, and William E. M. Lands, "Healthy Intakes of N-3 and N-6 Fatty
Acids: Estimations Considering Worldwide Diversity," *American Journal of
Clinical Nutrition* 83 (2006): 1483S–1493S.

128 **a gram a day has also been shown to be safe:** Berthold Koletzko,
Irene Cetin, and J. Thomas Brenna, "Dietary Fat Intakes for Pregnant and
Lactating Women," *British Journal of Nutrition* 98 (2007): 873–77.

128 **likely to be safe in amounts up to three times as high:** This is the
assessment of the Natural Medicines Comprehensive Database, an independent group. Before taking very large amounts of DHA, you should consult
with your physician, especially if you take blood thinners or anticoagulants.

130 **higher meat consumption is linked to heavier weights:** E. A. Spen-
cer, P. N. Appleby, G. K. Davey, and T. J. Key, "Diet and Body Mass
Index in 38000 Epic-Oxford Meat-Eaters, Fish-Eaters, Vegetarians and
Vegans," *International Journal of Obesity* 27 (2003): 728–34.

130 **women who eat larger amounts of meat:** See H. S. Kahn, L. M.
Tatham, C. Rodriguez, E. E. Calle, M. J. Thun, and C. W. Heath, Jr.,
"Stable Behaviors Associated with Adults' 10-Year Change in Body Mass
Index and Likelihood of Gain at the Waist," *American Journal of Public
Health* 87 (1997): 747–54. E. A. Spencer, P. N. Appleby, G. K. Davey, and
T. J. Key, "Diet and Body Mass Index in 38000 Epic-Oxford Meat-Eaters,
Fish-Eaters, Vegetarians and Vegans," *International Journal of Obesity* 27
(2003): 728–34. A. C. Vergnaud, T. Norat, D. Romaguera, T. Mouw,
A. M. May, N. Travier, et al., "Meat Consumption and Prospective
Weight Change in Participants of the Epic-Panacea Study," *American
Journal of Clinical Nutrition* 92 (2010): 398–407.

130 **Vegetarians tend to weigh less:** Timothy J. Key, Paul N. Appleby, and
Magdalena S. Rosell, "Health Effects of Vegetarian and Vegan Diets,"
Proceedings of the Nutrition Society 65 (2006): 35–41. Weight differences
for American women who consider themselves vegetarians and meat-
eaters are small.

130 **grass is rich in omega-3:** D. C. Rule, K. S. Broughton, S. M. Shellito,
and G. Maiorano, "Comparison of Muscle Fatty Acid Profiles and Cholesterol Concentrations of Bison, Beef Cattle, Elk, and Chicken," *Journal of
Animal Science* 80 (2002): 1202–11.

130 **in grass-fed beef:** See USDA National Nutrient Database and P. French,
C. Stanton, F. Lawless, E. G. O'Riordan, F. J. Monahan, P. J. Caffrey, and
A. P. Moloney, "Fatty Acid Composition, Including Conjugated Linoleic
Acid, of Intramuscular Fat from Steers Offered Grazed Grass, Grass Silage,
or Concentrate-Based Diets," *Journal of Animal Science* 78 (2000): 2849–55.

131 **wild game animals:** L. Cordain, B. A. Watkins, G. L. Flourant, M. Kehler, L. Rogers, and Y. Liu, "Fatty Acid Analysis of Wild Ruminant Tissues: Evolutionary Implications for Reducing Diet-Related Chronic Diseases," *European Journal of Clinical Nutrition* 56 (2002): 181–91.

131 **grass-fed beef has been found to be less likely to cause weight gain:** P. Legrand, B. Schmitt, J. Mourot, D. Catheline, G. Chesneau, et al., "The Consumption of Food Products from Linseed-Fed Animals Maintains Erythrocyte Omega-3 Fatty Acids in Obese Humans," *Lipids* 45 (2010): 11–19.

131 **significant amounts of DHA and EPA in their muscles:** Simba Nagahuedi, Jason T. Popesku, Vance L. Trudeau, and Jean-Michel Weber, "Mimicking the Natural Doping of Migrant Sandpipers in Sedentary Quails: Effects of Dietary N-3 Fatty Acids on Muscle Membranes and PPAR Expression," *Journal of Experimental Biology* 212 (2009): 1106–14.

131 **twice as much omega-3:** R. L. Husak, J. G. Sebranek, and K. Bregendahl, "A Survey of Commercially Available Broilers Marketed as Organic, Free-Range, and Conventional Broilers for Cooked Meat Yields, Meat Composition, and Relative Value," *Poultry Science* 87 (2008): 2367–76. P. I. P. Ponte, J. A. M. Prates, J. P. Crespo, D. G. Crespo, J. L. Mourão, S. P. Alves, R. J. B. Bessa, M. A. Chaveiro-Soares, L. T. Gama, L. M. A. Ferreira, and C. M. G. A. Fontes, "Restricting the Intake of a Cereal-Based Feed in Free-Range-Pastured Poultry: Effects on Performance and Meat Quality," *Poultry Science* 87 (2008): 2032–42.

132 **Eggs from chickens fed flaxseeds:** Mary E. Van Elswyk, "Nutritional and Physiological Effects of Flax Seed in Diets for Laying Fowl," *World's Poultry Science Journal* 53 (1997): 253–64.

133 **when fish is fried or coated in batter:** H. Chung, J. A. Nettleton, R. N. Lemaitre, R. G. Barr, M. Y. Tsai, R. P. Tracy, and D. S. Siscovick, "Frequency and Type of Seafood Consumed Influence Plasma (N-3) Fatty Acid Concentrations," *Journal of Nutrition* 138 (2008): 2422–27. M. I. Gladyshev, G. A. Gubanenko, N. N. Sushchik, S. M. Demirchieva, and G. S. Kalacheva, "Influence of Different Methods of Cooking of Hunchback Salmon on Contents of Polyunsaturated Fatty Acids," *Voprosy Pitaniia* 75 (2006): 47–50.

134–35 **Farmed fish may also have high levels of other pollutants:** See David W. Cole, Richard Cole, Steven J. Gaydos, Jon Gray, Greg Hyland, Mark L. Jacques, Nicole Powell-Dunford, Charu Sawhney, and William W. Au, "Aquaculture: Environmental, Toxicological, and Health Issues," *International Journal of Hygiene and Environmental Health* 212 (2009): 369–77.

135 **more omega-6 than wild-caught fish:** Kelly L. Weaver, Priscilla Ivester, Joshua A. Chilton, Martha D. Wilson, Prativa Pandey, and Floyd H. Chilton, "The Content of Favorable and Unfavorable Polyunsaturated Fatty Acids Found in Commonly Eaten Fish," *Journal of the American Dietetic Association* 108 (2008): 1178–85.

136 **Studies in Norwegian women:** M. B. Veierod, P. Laake, and D. S. Thelle, "Dietary Fat Intake and Risk of Lung Cancer: A Prospective Study of 51,452 Norwegian Men and Women," *European Journal of Cancer Prevention* 6 (1997): 540–49.

137 **dairy foods may help to reduce women's weights:** Michael B. Zemel, "The Role of Dairy Foods in Weight Management," *Journal of the American College of Nutrition* 24 (2005): 537S–546S. Gianvincenzo Barba and Paola Russo, "Dairy Foods, Dietary Calcium and Obesity: A Short Review of the Evidence," *Nutrition Metabolism & Cardiovascular Diseases* 16 (2006): 445–51.

137 **dairy foods are also linked to better general health:** Eva-Elisa Alvarez-León, Blanca Román-Viñas, and Lluís Serra-Majem, "Dairy Products and Health: A Review of the Epidemiological Evidence," *British Journal of Nutrition* 96, suppl. 1 (2006): S94–99. Michael B. Zemel, "Proposed Role of Calcium and Dairy Food Components in Weight Management and Metabolic Health," *Physician and Sportsmedicine* 37 (2009): 29–39. J. B. German, R. A. Gibson, R. M. Krauss, P. Nestel, B. Lamarche, W. A. van Staveren, J. M. Steijns, L. C. de Groot, A. L. Lock, and F. Destaillats, "A Reappraisal of the Impact of Dairy Foods and Milk Fat on Cardiovascular Disease Risk," *European Journal of Nutrition* 48 (2009): 191–203. L. Ebringer, M. Ferenck, and J. Krajcovic, "Beneficial Health Effects of Milk and Fermented Dairy Products—Review," *Folia Microbiologica* 53 (2008): 378–94.

137 **lower risks of broken bones:** Robert P. Heaney, "Dairy and Bone Health," *Journal of the American College of Nutrition* 28, suppl. 1 (2009): 82S–90S. D. Baran, A. Sorensen, J. Grimes, R. Lew, A. Karellas, B. Johnson, and J. Roche, "Dietary Modification with Dairy Products for Preventing Vertebral Bone Loss in Premenopausal Women: A Three-Year Prospective Study," *Journal of Clinical Endocrinology & Metabolism* 70 (1990): 264–70. Susanne Eriksson, Dan Mellstrom, and Birgitta Strandvik, "Fatty Acid Pattern in Serum Is Associated with Bone Mineralisation in Healthy 8-Year-Old Children," *British Journal of Nutrition* 102 (2009): 407–12. L. Esterle, J. P. Sabatier, F. Guillon-Metz, O. Walrant-Debray, G. Guaydier-Souquières, F. Jehan, and M. Garabédian, "Milk, Rather Than Other Foods, Is Associated with Vertebral Bone Mass and Circulating IGF-1 in Female Adolescents," *Osteoporosis International* 20 (2009): 567–75. Yannis Manios, George Moschonis, George Trovas, and George P. Lyritis, "Changes in Biochemical Indexes of Bone Metabolism and Bone Mineral

Density after a 12-Mo Dietary Intervention Program: The Postmenopausal Health Study," *American Journal of Clinical Nutrition* 86 (2007): 781–
89. George Moschonis, Ioanna Katsaroli, George P. Lyritis, and Yannis
Manios, "The Effects of a 30-Month Dietary Intervention on Bone Mineral Density: The Postmenopausal Health Study," *British Journal of Nutrition* 104 (2010): 100–107. Linda D. McCabe, Berdine R. Martin, George
P. McCabe, Conrad C. Johnston, Connie M. Weaver, and Munro Pea-
cock, "Dairy Intakes Affect Bone Density in the Elderly," *American Journal
of Clinical Nutrition* 80 (2004): 1066–74.

137 **Dairy foods also contain small amounts of natural trans fats**:
Arunabh Bhattacharya, Jameela Banu, Mizanur Rahman, Jennifer Causey,
and Gabriel Fernandes, "Biological Effects of Conjugated Linoleic Acids in
Health and Disease," *Journal of Nutritional Biochemistry* 17 (2006): 789–810.

137 **A recent extensive review:** P. W. Siri-Tarino, Q. Sun, F. B. Hu, and
R. M. Krauss, "Meta-Analysis of Prospective Cohort Studies Evaluating
the Association of Saturated Fat with Cardiovascular Disease," *American
Journal of Clinical Nutrition* 91 (2010): 535–46. See also Marion G. Volk,
"An Examination of the Evidence Supporting the Association of Dietary
Cholesterol and Saturated Fats with Serum Cholesterol and Development
of Coronary Heart Disease," *Alternative Medicine Review* 12 (2007):
228–45. F. B. Hu, J. E. Manson, and W. C. Willett, "Types of Dietary Fat
and Risk of Coronary Heart Disease: A Critical Review," *Journal of the
American College of Nutrition* 20 (2001): 5–19. L. Hooper, C. D. Summer-
bell, J. P. Higgins, R. L. Thompson, G. Clements, N. Capps, S. Davey,
R. A. Riemersma, and S. Ebrahim, "Reduced or Modified Dietary Fat
for Preventing Cardiovascular Disease," *Cochrane Database of Systematic
Reviews* (2001): CD002137.

138 **Nor is saturated fat intake connected to cholesterol:** C. Bolton-
Smith, M. Woodward, W. C. Smith, and H. Tunstall-Pedoe, "Dietary
and Non-Dietary Predictors of Serum Total and HDL-Cholesterol in
Men and Women: Results from the Scottish Heart Health Study," *International Journal of Epidemiology* 20 (1991): 95–104. H. Kesteloot, "Cardiovascular Risk Factors and Mortality in Women," *Herz* 12 (1987): 248–54.

138 **omega-3 in the diet is much more beneficial:** M. F. Oliver, "It Is
More Important to Increase the Intake of Unsaturated Fats Than to
Decrease the Intake of Saturated Fats: Evidence from Clinical Trials
Relating to Ischemic Heart Disease," *American Journal of Clinical Nutrition*
66 (1997): 980S–86S.

138 **Vitamin D deficiency seems to be a growing problem:** Anne C. Looker,
Christine M. Pfeiffer, David A. Lacher, Rosemary L. Schleicher, Mary
Frances Picciano, and Elizabeth A. Yetley, "Serum 25-Hydroxyvitamin D
Status of the US Population: 1988–1994 Compared with 2000–2004,"
American Journal of Clinical Nutrition 88 (2008): 1519–27.

138 **make your own vitamin D:** See Michael J. Holick, *The Vitamin D Solution: A 3-Step Strategy to Cure Our Most Common Health Problem* (New York: Hudson Street Press, 2010).

139 **heavier women have lower fiber intake:** See for example M. A. Alfieri, J. Pomerleau, D. M. Grace, and L. Anderson, "Fiber Intake of Normal Weight, Moderately Obese and Severely Obese Subjects," *Obesity Research* 3 (1995): 541–47. Jaimie N. Davis, Valerie A. Hodges, and M. Beth Gillham, "Normal-Weight Adults Consume More Fiber and Fruit than Their Age- and Height-Matched Overweight/Obese Counterparts," *Journal of the American Dietetic Association* 106 (2006): 833–40.

139 **women with higher fiber intakes tend to live longer:** Yikyung Park, Amy F. Subar, Albert Hollenbeck, and Arthur Schatzkin, "Dietary Fiber Intake and Mortality in the NIH-AARP Diet and Health Study," *Archives of Internal Medicine* posted online February 14 (2011). S. Todd, M. Woodward, H. Tunstall-Pedoe, and C. Bolton-Smith, "Dietary Antioxidant Vitamins and Fiber in the Etiology of Cardiovascular Disease and All-Causes Mortality: Results from the Scottish Heart Health Study," *American Journal of Epidemiology* 150 (1999): 1073–80.

139 **Fiber supplements may also help to lower women's weights:** Sebely Pal, Alireza Khossousi, Colin Binns, Satvinder Dhaliwal, and Vanessa Ellis, "The Effect of a Fibre Supplement Compared to a Healthy Diet on Body Composition, Lipids, Glucose, Insulin and Other Metabolic Syndrome Risk Factors in Overweight and Obese Individuals," *British Journal of Nutrition* 105 (2011): 90–100.

140 **Potato chips made with lard:** The Utz potato chip company sells chips made with lard for those who would like to taste the difference.

140 **total amount of vegetables:** T. A. Ledoux, M. D. Hingle, and T. Baranowski, "Relationship of Fruit and Vegetable Intake with Adiposity: A Systematic Review," *Obesity Reviews* July 14 [e-publication ahead of print] (2010).

140 **more fruit in the diet has also been linked with lower weights:** S. Alinia, O. Hels, and I. Tetens, "The Potential Association Between Fruit Intake and Body Weight—a Review," *Obesity Reviews* 10 (2009): 639–47.

140 **nutrients in American women's blood:** See also Tracy L. Burrows, Janet M. Warren, Kim Colyvas, Manohar L. Garg, and Clare E. Collins, "Validation of Overweight Children's Fruit and Vegetable Intake Using Plasma Carotenoids," *Obesity* 17 (2009): 162–68. Weiwen Chai, Shannon M. Conroy, Gertraud Maskarinec, Adrian A. Franke, Ian S. Pagano, and Robert V. Cooney, "Associations Between Obesity and Serum Lipid-Soluble Micronutrients Among Premenopausal Women," *Nutrition Research* 30 (2010): 227–32. A. Drewnowski, C. L. Rock, S. A. Henderson, A. B. Shore, C. Fischler, P. Galan, P. Preziosi, and S. Hercberg, "Serum Beta-Carotene and Vitamin C as Biomarkers of Vegetable and Fruit

Intakes in a Community-Based Sample of French Adults," *American Journal of Clinical Nutrition* 65 (1997): 1796–1802.

140 **orange carotenes and yellow xanthins:** Alpha- and beta-carotene, alpha-cryptoxanthin, zeaxanthin, lutein (a xanthophyll).

141 **high in beta-carotene reduce the risk of cancer:** World Cancer Research Fund and the American Institute for Cancer Research, *Food, Nutrition and the Prevention of Cancer: A Global Perspective* (Washington D.C.: American Institute for Cancer Research, 1997).

141 **beta-carotene supplements do not:** Goran Bjelakovic, Dimitrinka Nikolova, Lise Lotte Gluud, Rosa G. Simonetti, and Christian Gluud, "Mortality in Randomized Trials of Antioxidant Supplements for Primary and Secondary Prevention: Systematic Review and Meta-Analysis," *Journal of the American Medical Association* 297 (2007): 842–57.

141 **Beginning a meal with a salad:** Barbara J. Rolls, Liane S. Roe, and Jennifer S. Meengs, "Salad and Satiety: Energy Density and Portion Size of a First-Course Salad Affect Energy Intake at Lunch," *Journal of the American Dietetic Association* 104 (2004): 1570–76.

142 **chocolate . . . may help to reduce weight:** Naoko Matsui, Ryoichi Ito, Eisaku Nishimura, Mariko Yoshikawa, Masatoshi Kato, Masanori Kamei, Haruki Shibata, Ichiro Matsumoto, Keiko Abe, and Shuichi Hashizume, "Ingested Cocoa Can Prevent High-Fat Diet-Induced Obesity by Regulating the Expression of Genes for Fatty Acid Metabolism," *Nutrition* 21 (2005): 594–601. C. E. O'Neil, V. L. Fulgoni III, and T. A. Nicklas, "Candy Consumption Was Not Associated with Body Weight Measures, Risk Factors for Cardiovascular Disease, or Metabolic Syndrome in US Adults: NHANES 1999–2004," *Nutrition Research* 31 (2011): 122–30.

142 **feeling of being satisfied:** Will Clower, *The Fat Fallacy* (New York: Three Rivers Press, 2003).

142 **decrease the risk of heart disease, high blood pressure, inflammation, and cancer:** Roberto Corti, Andreas J. Flammer, Norman K. Hollenberg, and Thomas F. Lüscher, "Cocoa and Cardiovascular Health," *Circulation* 119 (2009): 1433–41. Monica Galleano, Patricia I. Oteiza, and Cesar G. Fraga, "Cocoa, Chocolate, and Cardiovascular Disease," *Journal of Cardiovascular Pharmacology* 54 (2009): 483–90. Carlo Selmi, Claudio A. Cocchi, Mario Lanfredini, Carl L. Keen, and M. Eric Gershwin, "Chocolate at Heart: The Anti-Inflammatory Impact of Cocoa Flavanols," *Molecular Nutrition & Food Research* 52 (2008): 1340–48. Emma Ramiro-Puig and Margarida Castell, "Cocoa: Antioxidant and Immunomodulator," *British Journal of Nutrition* 101 (2009): 931–40. Gertraud Maskarinec, "Cancer Protective Properties of Cocoa: A Review of the Epidemiologic Evidence," *Nutrition & Cancer* 61 (2009): 573–79.

144 **lighter American women actually report *more* sugar:** C. J. Lewis, Y. K. Park, P. B. Dexter, and E. A. Yetley, "Nutrient Intakes and Body

Weights of Persons Consuming High and Moderate Levels of Added Sugars," *Journal of the American Dietetic Association* 92 (1992): 708–13. J. I. Macdiarmid, A. Vail, J. E. Cade, and J. E. Blundell, "The Sugar-Fat Relationship Revisited: Differences in Consumption Between Men and Women of Varying BMI," *International Journal of Obesity & Related Metabolic Disorders: Journal of the International Association for the Study of Obesity* 22 (1998): 1053–61. C. Bolton-Smith, "Intake of Sugars in Relation to Fatness and Micronutrient Adequacy," *International Journal of Obesity & Related Metabolic Disorders: Journal of the International Association for the Study of Obesity* 20, suppl. 2 (1996): S31–33. J. O. Hill and A. M. Prentice, "Sugar and Body Weight Regulation," *American Journal of Clinical Nutrition* 62 (1995): 264S–73S; discussion 73S–74S. Wim H. M. Saris, "Sugars, Energy Metabolism, and Body Weight Control," *American Journal of Clinical Nutrition* 78 (2003): 850S–57S. S. H. Vermunt, W. J. Pasman, G. Schaafsma, and A. F. Kardinaal, "Effects of Sugar Intake on Body Weight: A Review," *Obesity Reviews* 4 (2003): 91–99. David Benton, "The Plausibility of Sugar Addiction and Its Role in Obesity and Eating Disorders," *Clinical Nutrition* 29 (2010): 288–303. M. A. van Baak and A. Astrup, "Consumption of Sugars and Body Weight," *Obesity Reviews* 10, suppl. 1 (2009): 9–23.

144 **studies that use chemical methods to monitor sugar:** Karin Vagstrand, Anna Karin Lindroos, Dowen Birkhed, and Yvonne Linne, "Associations between Salivary Bacteria and Reported Sugar Intake and Their Relationship with Body Mass Index in Women and Their Adolescent Children," *Public Health Nutrition* 11 (2008): 341–48. Sheila Bingham, Robert Luben, Ailsa Welch, Natasa Tasevska, Nick Wareham, and Kay Tee Khaw, "Epidemiologic Assessment of Sugars Consumption Using Biomarkers: Comparisons of Obese and Nonobese Individuals in the European Prospective Investigation of Cancer Norfolk," *Cancer Epidemiology, Biomarkers & Prevention* 16 (2007): 1651–54.

144 **sugar-sweetened beverages:** Colin D. Rehm, Thomas D. Matte, Gretchen Van Wye, Candace Young, and Thomas R. Frieden, "Demographic and Behavioral Factors Associated with Daily Sugar-Sweetened Soda Consumption in New York City Adults," *Journal of Urban Health* 85 (2008): 375–85. Katja Nissinen, Vera Mikkilä, Satu Männistö, Marjaana Lahti-Koski, Leena Räsänen, Jorma Viikari, and Olli T. Raitakari, "Sweets and Sugar-Sweetened Soft Drink Intake in Childhood in Relation to Adult BMI and Overweight: The Cardiovascular Risk in Young Finns Study," *Public Health Nutrition* 12 (2009): 2018–26. Emily Wolff, and Michael L. Dansinger, "Soft Drinks and Weight Gain: How Strong Is the Link?" *Medscape Journal of Medicine* 10 (2008): 189. Vasanti S. Malik, Matthias B. Schulze, and Frank B. Hu, "Intake of Sugar-Sweetened Beverages and Weight Gain: A Systematic Review," *American Journal of Clinical Nutrition* 84 (2006): 274–88.

144 **women who use artificial sweeteners tend to gain more weight:**
Richard D. Mattes and Barry M. Popkin, "Nonnutritive Sweetener Consumption in Humans: Effects on Appetite and Food Intake and Their Putative Mechanisms," *American Journal of Clinical Nutrition* 89 (2009): 1–14.
F. Bellisle and C. Perez, "Low-Energy Substitutes for Sugars and Fats in
the Human Diet: Impact on Nutritional Regulation," *Neuroscience & Biobe-
havioral Reviews* 18 (1994): 197–205. Qing Yang, "Gain Weight By 'Going
Diet?' Artificial Sweeteners and the Neurobiology of Sugar Cravings: Neuroscience 2010," *Yale Journal of Biology & Medicine* 83 (2010): 101–8.

146 **low-carb diets have not proven to be any better:** Michael L. Dan-
singer, Joi Augustin Gleason, John L. Griffith, Harry P. Selker, and Ernst J.
Schaefer, "Comparison of the Atkins, Ornish, Weight Watchers, and Zone
Diets for Weight Loss and Heart Disease Risk Reduction: A Randomized
Trial," *Journal of the American Medical Association* 293 (2005): 43–53. Chris-
topher D. Gardner, Alexandre Kiazand, Sofiya Alhassan, Soowon Kim,
Randall S. Stafford, et al., "Comparison of the Atkins, Zone, Ornish, and
Learn Diets for Change in Weight and Related Risk Factors Among Over-
weight Premenopausal Women: The A to Z Weight Loss Study: A Ran-
domized Trial," *Journal of the American Medical Association* 297 (2007):
969–77. Helen Truby, Sue Baic, Anne deLooy, Kenneth R. Fox,
M. Barbara E. Livingstone, et al., "Randomised Controlled Trial of Four
Commercial Weight Loss Programmes in the UK: Initial Findings from
the BBC 'Diet Trials,'" *British Medical Journal* 332 (2006): 1309–14.

146 **glycemic index:** See Glenn A. Gaesser, "Carbohydrate Quantity and
Quality in Relation to Body Mass Index," *Journal of the American Dietetic
Association* 107 (2007): 1768–80. Marta Rossi, Cristina Bosetti, Renato
Talamini, Pagona Lagiou, Eva Negri, Silvia Franceschi, and Carlo La Vec-
chia, "Glycemic Index and Glycemic Load in Relation to Body Mass
Index and Waist to Hip Ratio," *European Journal of Nutrition* 49 (2010):
459–64.

147 **lower weights and less waist fat in women with more olive oil:**
Nadiah Moussavi, Victor Gavino, and Olivier Receveur, "Is Obesity
Related to the Type of Dietary Fatty Acids? An Ecological Study," *Public
Health Nutrition* 11 (2008): 1149–55. F. Soriguer, M. C. Almaraz, M. S.
Ruiz-de-Adana, I. Esteva, F. Linares, J. M. Garcia-Almeida, S. Morcillo,
E. Garcia-Escobar, G. Olveira-Fuster, and G. Rojo-Martinez, "Incidence
of Obesity Is Lower in Persons Who Consume Olive Oil," *European Jour-
nal of Clinical Nutrition* 63 (2009): 1371–74. Maria Garaulet, F. Perez-
Llamas, M. Perez-Ayala, P. Martinez, F. S. de Medina, F. J. Tebar, and
S. Zamora, "Site-Specific Differences in the Fatty Acid Composition of
Abdominal Adipose Tissue in an Obese Population from a Mediterranean
Area," *American Journal of Clinical Nutrition* 74 (2001): 585–91.

150 **a favorable effect of nuts on weight:** Richard D. Mattes and Mark L. Dreher, "Nuts and Healthy Body Weight Maintenance Mechanisms," *Asia Pacific Journal of Clinical Nutrition* 19 (2010): 137–41. Richard D. Mattes, Penny M. Kris-Etherton, and Gary D. Foster, "Impact of Peanuts and Tree Nuts on Body Weight and Healthy Weight Loss in Adults," *Journal of Nutrition* 138 (2008): 1741S–45S. Maira Bes-Rastrollo, Nicole M. Wedick, Miguel Angel Martinez-Gonzalez, Tricia Y. Li, Laura Sampson, and Frank B. Hu, "Prospective Study of Nut Consumption, Long-Term Weight Change, and Obesity Risk in Women," *American Journal of Clinical Nutrition* 89 (2009): 1913–19.

150 **nuts may be beneficial to health:** G. E. Fraser, "Associations Between Diet and Cancer, Ischemic Heart Disease, and All-Cause Mortality in Non-Hispanic White California Seventh-Day Adventists," *American Journal of Clinical Nutrition* 70 (1999): 532S–38S. Ross Grant, Ayse Bilgin, Carol Zeuschner, Trish Guy, Robyn Pearce, Bevan Hokin, and John Ashton, "The Relative Impact of a Vegetable-Rich Diet on Key Markers of Health in a Cohort of Australian Adolescents," *Asia Pacific Journal of Clinical Nutrition* 17 (2008): 107–15. F. Lavedrine, D. Zmirou, A. Ravel, F. Balducci, and J. Alary, "Blood Cholesterol and Walnut Consumption: A Cross-Sectional Survey in France," *Preventive Medicine* 28 (1999): 333–39. Sabaté Joan and Yen Ang, "Nuts and Health Outcomes: New Epidemiologic Evidence," *American Journal of Clinical Nutrition* 89 (2009): 1643S–48S. Stephen D. Nash and David T. Nash, "Nuts as Part of a Healthy Cardiovascular Diet," *Current Atherosclerosis Reports* 10 (2008): 529–35.

150 **an especially good choice for snacks:** Anna-Lena Claesson, Gunilla Holm, Asa Ernersson, Torbjorn Lindstrom, and Fredrik H. Nystrom, "Two Weeks of Overfeeding with Candy, but Not Peanuts, Increases Insulin Levels and Body Weight," *Scandinavian Journal of Clinical & Laboratory Investigation* 69 (2009): 598–605.

153 **Michael Pollan's suggestion:** Michael Pollan, *In Defense of Food* (New York: Penguin, 2008).

156 **unwanted calories are more likely to be stored:** T. Yanover and W. P. Sacco, "Eating Beyond Satiety and Body Mass Index," *Eating & Weight Disorders* 13 (2008): 119–28.

158 **timing of your meals to set your tenty-four-hour biological clock:** J. Mendoza, "Circadian Clocks: Setting Time by Food," *Journal of Neuroendocrinology* 19 (2007): 127–37.

158 **disrupting your normal clock cycle:** L. K. Fonken, J. L. Workman, J. C. Walton, Z. M. Weil, J. S. Morris, A. Haim, and R. J. Nelson, "Light at Night Increases Body Mass by Shifting the Time of Food Intake," *Proceedings of the National Academy of Sciences of the United States of America* 107 (2010): 18664–69 John M. de Castro, "When, How Much and What

Foods Are Eaten Are Related to Total Daily Food Intake," *British Journal of Nutrition* 102 (2009): 1228–37.

158 **women eating breakfast has been declining:** P. S. Haines, D. K. Guilkey, and B. M. Popkin, "Trends in Breakfast Consumption of U.S. Adults Between 1965 and 1991," *Journal of the American Dietetic Association* 96 (1996): 464–70.

158 **women who skip a morning meal:** Margaret Ashwell, "An Examination of the Relationship Between Breakfast, Weight and Shape," *British Journal of Nursing* 19 (2010): 1155–59.

159 **eat late at night tend to weigh more:** G. S. Andersen, A. J. Stunkard, T. I. Sorensen, L. Petersen, B. L. Heitmann, "Night Eating and Weight Change in Middle-Aged Men and Women," *International Journal of Obesity* 28 (2004): 1338–43. Marci E. Gluck, Colleen A. Venti, Arline D. Salbe, and Jonathan Krakoff, "Nighttime Eating: Commonly Observed and Related to Weight Gain in an Inpatient Food Intake Study," *American Journal of Clinical Nutrition* 88 (2008): 900–905.

159 **an experiment done at a Philadelphia cinema:** Brian Wansink and Junyong Kim, "Bad Popcorn in Big Buckets: Portion Size Can Influence Intake as Much as Taste," *Journal of Nutrition Education & Behavior* 37 (2005): 242–45.

159 **People given these secretly replenishing bowls:** Brian Wansink, James E. Painter, and Jill North, "Bottomless Bowls: Why Visual Cues of Portion Size May Influence Intake," *Obesity Research* 13 (2005): 93–100.

160 **women eat more when they are offered larger portions:** Tanja V. E. Kral, "Effects on Hunger and Satiety, Perceived Portion Size and Pleasantness of Taste of Varying the Portion Size of Foods: A Brief Review of Selected Studies," *Appetite* 46 (2006): 103–5.

160 **dish out larger portion sizes:** Christina Berg, Georgios Lappas, Alicja Wolk, Elisabeth Strandhagen, Kjell Toren, Annika Rosengren, Dag Thelle, and Lauren Lissner, "Eating Patterns and Portion Size Associated with Obesity in a Swedish Population," *Appetite* 52 (2009): 21–26. Kyle S. Burger, Mark Kern, and Karen J. Coleman, "Characteristics of Self-Selected Portion Size in Young Adults," *Journal of the American Dietetic Association* 107 (2007): 611–18.

160 **little evidence that they cut back in calories:** Mary T. Kelly, Julie M. W. Wallace, Paula J. Robson, Kirsten L. Rennie, Robert W. Welch, Mary P. Hannon-Fletcher, Sarah Brennan, Adrian Fletcher, and M. B. E. Livingstone, "Increased Portion Size Leads to a Sustained Increase in Energy Intake over 4 D in Normal-Weight and Overweight Men and Women," *British Journal of Nutrition* 102 (2009): 470–77.

161 **having nuts for snacks can lower weight:** Anna-Lena Claesson, Gunilla Holm, Asa Ernersson, Torbjorn Lindstrom, and Fredrik H. Nystrom, "Two Weeks of Overfeeding with Candy, but Not Peanuts,

Increases Insulin Levels and Body Weight," *Scandinavian Journal of Clinical & Laboratory Investigation* 69 (2009): 598–605.

161 **larger number of small meals:** Andre M. Toschke, Helmut Kuchenhoff, Berthold Koletzko, and Rudiger von Kries, "Meal Frequency and Childhood Obesity," *Obesity Research* 13 (2005): 1932–38.

162 **countries with data on soft drinks:** Data from Global Market Information Database: www.euromonitor.com/.

163 **Institute of Medicine:** "Dietary Reference Intakes: Water, Potassium, Sodium, Chloride, and Sulfate," 2004, http://iom.edu/Reports/2004/Dietary-Reference-Intakes-Water-Potassium-Sodium-Chloride-and-Sulfate.aspx.

163 **water, especially before a meal, may help to prevent weight gain:** E. A. Dennis, A. L. Dengo, D. L. Comber, K. D. Flack, J. Savla, K. P. Davy, and B. M. Davy, "Water Consumption Increases Weight Loss During a Hypocaloric Diet Intervention in Middle-Aged and Older Adults," *Obesity* 18 (2010): 300–307. Ashima K. Kant, Barry I. Graubard, and Elizabeth A. Atchison, "Intakes of Plain Water, Moisture in Foods and Beverages, and Total Water in the Adult US Population—Nutritional, Meal Pattern, and Body Weight Correlates: National Health and Nutrition Examination Surveys 1999–2006," *American Journal of Clinical Nutrition* 90 (2009): 655–63. Jodi D. Stookey, Florence Constant, Barry M. Popkin, and Christopher D. Gardner, "Drinking Water Is Associated with Weight Loss in Overweight Dieting Women Independent of Diet and Activity," *Obesity* 16 (2008): 2481–88.

163 **lower weights with modest amounts of alcohol:** Martin R. Yeomans, "Alcohol, Appetite and Energy Balance: Is Alcohol Intake a Risk Factor for Obesity?" *Physiology & Behavior* 100 (2010): 82–89.

163 **wine has the most benefit:** Esther Lukasiewicz, Louise I. Mennen, Sandrine Bertrais, Nathalie Arnault, Paul Preziosi, Pilar Galan, and Serge Hercberg, "Alcohol Intake in Relation to Body Mass Index and Waist-to-Hip Ratio: The Importance of Type of Alcoholic Beverage," *Public Health Nutrition* 8 (2005): 315–20.

163 **health benefits:** M. A. Collins, E. J. Neafsey, K. J. Mukamal, M. O. Gray, D. A. Parks, D. K. Das, and R. J. Korthuis, "Alcohol in Moderation, Cardioprotection, and Neuroprotection: Epidemiological Considerations and Mechanistic Studies," *Alcoholism: Clinical and Experimental Research* 33 (2009): 206–19.

163 **alcohol . . . increasing omega-3:** R. di Giuseppe, M. de Lorgeril, P. Salen, F. Laporte, A. Di Castelnuovo, V. Krogh, A. Siani, J. Arnout, F. P. Cappuccio, M. van Dongen, M. B. Donati, G. de Gaetano, L. Iacoviello, "Alcohol Consumption and N-3 Polyunsaturated Fatty Acids in Healthy Men and Women from 3 European Populations," *American Journal of Clinical Nutrition* 89 (2009): 354–62.

164 **Americans walk less:** David R. Bassett, Jr., Holly R. Wyatt, Helen Thompson, John C. Peters, and James O. Hill, "Pedometer-Measured Physical Activity and Health Behaviors in U.S. Adults," *Medicine and Science in Sports and Exercise* 42 (2010): 1819–25.

164 **more trips by bicycle or on foot:** John Pucher, Ralph Buehler, David R. Bassett, and Andrew L. Dannenberg, "Walking and Cycling to Health: A Comparative Analysis of City, State, and International Data," *American Journal of Public Health* 100 (2010): 1986–92.

164 **walks for at least thirty minutes a day:** John Pucher, Ralph Buehler, Dafna Merom, and Adrian Bauman, "Walking and Cycling in the United States, 2001–2009: Evidence from the National Household Travel Surveys," *American Journal of Public Health* published online May 6 (2011): doi:10.2105/AJPH.010.300067.

164 **exercise to help them lose weight:** The weight change in women who increased exercise is from the NHANES 2007–8.

164 **ten thousand steps:** Patrick L. Schneider, David R. Bassett, Jr., Dixie L. Thompson, Nicolaas P. Pronk, and Kenneth M. Bielak, "Effects of a 10,000 Steps Per Day Goal in Overweight Adults," *American Journal of Health Promotion* 21 (2006): 85–9.

165 **dishes we now serve at dinner are ready-to-eat:** NPD Group, "America's Hurried Lifestyle Has Greatest Impact on Eating Behaviors over Last 30 Years," NPD Press Release, October 18, 2010.

165 **prepared foods in the diets of today's young adult women:** Nicole I. Larson, Cheryl L. Perry, Mary Story, and Dianne Neumark-Sztainer, "Food Preparation by Young Adults Is Associated with Better Diet Quality," *Journal of the American Dietetic Association* 106 (2006): 2001–7.

165 **cost per calorie in a diet of convenience foods:** Andrew J. McDermott and Mark B. Stephens, "Cost of Eating: Whole Foods Versus Convenience Foods in a Low-Income Model," *Family Medicine* 42 (2010): 280–84.

165–166 **most of those who rely on convenience foods agree**: NPD Group, "Convenience Drives Daily Food Choices for Most American Adults—but in Different Ways, Reports NPD," NPD Press Release, January 26, 2010.

169 **researchers from Yale University:** Marlene B. Schwartz, Lenny R. Vartanian, Brian A. Nosek, and Kelly D. Brownell, "The Influence of One's Own Body Weight on Implicit and Explicit Anti-Fat Bias," *Obesity* 14 (3) (2006): 440–47.

170 **luck of the draw:** Chris Cotsapas, Elizabeth K. Speliotes, Ida J. Hatoum, Danielle M. Greenawalt, Radu Dobrin, Pek Y. Lum, et al., "Common Body Mass Index–Associated Variants Confer Risk of Extreme Obesity," *Human Molecular Genetics* 18 (2009): 3502–7.

173 **those differences are determined by the genes:** C. M. Carmichael and
M. McGue, "A Cross-Sectional Examination of Height, Weight, and Body
Mass Index in Adult Twins," *Journals of Gerontology Series A—Biological Sci-
ences & Medical Sciences* 50 (1995): B237–44.

173 **how thick their bones are:** D. Karasik, N. A. Shimabuku, Y. Zhou, Y.
Zhang, L. A. Cupples, D. P. Kiel, and S. Demissie, "A Genome Wide
Linkage Scan of Metacarpal Size and Geometry in the Framingham
Study," *American Journal of Human Biology* 20 (2008): 663–70.

173 **width of your shoulders and hip bones:** Alaitz Poveda, Aline Jelen-
kovic, Charles Susanne, and Esther Rebato, "Genetic Contribution to
Variation in Body Configuration in Belgian Nuclear Families: A Closer
Look at Body Lengths and Circumferences," *Collegium Antropologicum* 34
(2010): 515–23.

174 **how much fat you have is also strongly governed by your genes:**
M. S. Faith, A. Pietrobelli, C. Nunez, M. Heo, S. B. Heymsfield, and D.
B. Allison, "Evidence for Independent Genetic Influences on Fat Mass and
Body Mass Index in a Pediatric Twin Sample," *Pediatrics* 104 (1999): 61–
67. T. Rice, C. Bouchard, L. Perusse, and D. C. Rao, "Familial Cluster-
ing of Multiple Measures of Adiposity and Fat Distribution in the Quebec
Family Study: A Trivariate Analysis of Percent Body Fat, Body Mass
Index, and Trunk-to-Extremity Skinfold Ratio," *International Journal of
Obesity* 19 (1995): 902–8.

175 **fat in their lower body or their waist:** D. G. Carey, T. V. Nguyen,
L. V. Campbell, D. J. Chisholm, and P. Kelly, "Genetic Influences on
Central Abdominal Fat: A Twin Study," *International Journal of Obesity* 20
(1996): 722–26.

199 ***As Nature Made Him:*** John Colapinto, *As Nature Made Him: The Boy Who
Was Raised as a Girl* (New York: HarperCollins, 2000).

200 **usually begin regaining weight over time:** M. D. Kofman, M. R.
Lent, and C. Swencionis, "Maladaptive Eating Patterns, Quality of Life,
and Weight Outcomes Following Gastric Bypass: Results of an Internet
Survey," *Obesity* 18 (2010): 1938–43. Loren Dalcanale, Claudia P.
Oliveira, Joel Faintuch, Monize A. Nogueira, Patricia Rondo, Vic Lima,
et al., "Long-Term Nutritional Outcome After Gastric Bypass," *Obesity
Surgery* 20 (2010): 181–87. Meena Shah, Vinaya Simha, and Abhimanyu
Garg, "Review: Long-Term Impact of Bariatric Surgery on Body Weight,
Comorbidities, and Nutritional Status," *Journal of Clinical Endocrinology &
Metabolism* 91 (2006): 4223–31. Dani O. Magro, Bruno Geloneze, Regis
Delfini, Bruna Contini Pareja, Francisco Callejas, and Jos C. Pareja,
"Long-Term Weight Regain after Gastric Bypass: A 5-Year Prospective
Study," *Obesity Surgery* 18 (2008): 648–51.

INDEX